Sexually Transmitted Infections

Anita Weston
RGN, MSc, Cert. Ed, Cert. Counselling Skills,
PG Cert. Applied Research Methodologies

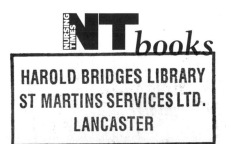

Acknowledgements

I am grateful to everyone at the Nursing Times for their encouragement and support with this venture, especially Janet Gillan who commissioned the two sexual health series, Alison Whyte, Brian Booth, Martin Vousden and Simon Seljeflot.

Thanks also to Professor Robert Pratt, Director of the Centre for Sexual Health and HIV Studies at the Wolfson Institute of Health Sciences, Thames Valley University, London, who has been a constant source of support and inspiration to me throughout my career in sexual health, and continues to be so.

Thanks to Debbie Baker, Nurse Practitioner, whose commitment to caring for people with STIs, and the standard of care she delivers to those people, has inspired many nurses, including myself. Thanks to Val Driver for administrative support and patience, and finally, thanks to all our students, past and present, of the ENB 275 and ENB 276 courses for their enthusiasm and support. It is to them that I dedicate this book.

Names of patients in case studies have been changed.

First published 1999 by Nursing Times Books
Emap Healthcare Ltd, part of Emap Business Communications
Greater London House
Hampstead Road
London NW1 7EJ

Text © 1999 Emap Healthcare Ltd

Cover illustration:
Hyphae and spores of *Candida albicans* in a vaginal smear by Gram stain, © Anita Weston

Printed and bound in Great Britain by Drogher Press, Christchurch, Dorset

British Library cataloguing in Publication Data
A catalogue record for this book is available from the British Library.

ISBN: 1902499093

Contents

Biographies

Sue Chard, GN, ENB 900/1, 225, 934

Sue is the Senior Research Sister in GUM/HIV at the St Stephen's Centre at The Chelsea and Westminster Hospital. For the past six years she has taught part-time on the ENB 275/6 course "Caring for persons with Genito-urinary infections and related problems" and the ENB 934 "Care and management of people with HIV disease", at Thames Valley University (previously at the Riverside College of Health Studies). She also teaches about contraception and genito-urinary and HIV-related issues in local Secondary Schools in Kensington and Chelsea, London, and she has presented at international conferences.

Annabel Davis RGN, PGDip Health Promotion, ENB 934, 276, 870

Annabel is a Health Promotion Advisor for Schools and Young People in Kensington and Chelsea and Westminster Health Authority Department of Health Promotion. She has a background in sexual health, having worked in GUM clinics across London for four years. During this time she was involved in shaping young people's sexual health services and developing and delivering relationships and sex education in schools. While on placement as a postgraduate student at Camden Department of Health Promotion, Annabel worked on a project which aims to support the health and social care needs of refugees and asylum seekers from the Horn of Africa. In her free time, Annabel undertakes some freelance sexual health work; lecturing; speaking at conferences; writing articles for the *Nursing Times* and supporting the curriculum development of ENB courses.

Marsh Gelbart, RGN, BA, MA

Marsh qualified in Sheffield in 1981 and has worked as a nurse in Britain and abroad. He worked at the London Lighthouse in HIV/AIDS as a primary nurse for five years and is currently working as a health adviser at the John Hunter Clinic, HIV/GUM Directorate, at the Chelsea and Westminster NHS Trust, London.

Pippa Greer RGN, ENB 275, 934, 901 and 962

Pippa is a Nurse Practitioner working for the Praed Street Project. This project works with all women associated with the sex industry and is based at St Mary's Hospital in London. As well as her role as Nurse Practitioner she is also involved with the drop-in and the outreach work offered by the service.

Chris McGlynn, RGN, Dip. H.E., ENB 275, 934 and 901

Chris is Senior Sister for Genito-urinary Medicine and Sexual Health at The Royal Hospitals NHS Trust and is responsible for nursing staff at the Ambrose King Centre at the Royal London Hospital, Whitechapel and Barts Sexual Health Centre at St Bartholemew's Hospital. She teaches pre-registration and post-registration students about sexual health issues and STIs.

Sandy Nelson, BEd, MA Psychotherapy

Sandy is a Senior Lecturer in Sexual Health in the School of Community and Social Policy at the Wolfson Institute of Health Sciences at Thames Valley University, London. She teaches on various courses about human sexuality counselling and clinical supervision and is module leader for the Foundation Programme in Family Planning and Sexual Health Care. She also has a small, private, psychotherapy practice and does some freelance training and organisational consulting.

Heledd Nicholas

Heledd is Senior Nurse at the Caldecot Centre, a department of sexual health based at King's Healthcare Trust in south London and one of the busiest GUM clinics in the country.

Since specialising in GUM nursing in 1986, Heledd has also worked as a Health Adviser at the Middlesex Hospital in London and Sydney Hospital in Australia. During this time she was in the core team that set up one of the first counselling and information services for people with HIV infection. This service later became a prototype for other initiatives, both nationally and internationally, in the early years of dealing with HIV.

Subsequently, she initiated outreach projects aimed to disseminate sexual health education to hard-to-reach vulnerable groups such as prostitutes, the homeless and those in prison. In the mid-1990s she was actively involved in setting up a forensic sexual health service, in collaboration with the London Metropolitan Police, for people who had been sexually assaulted or raped.

Caroline Smales, RGN; Bsc Nursing; Cert Ed; Diploma in Infection Control; ENB 50I

Caroline is a Senior Lecturer in the School of Health, Community and Social Policy at the Wolfson Institute of Health Science, Thames Valley University. She has developed extensive knowledge and skills in the field of infectious diseases nursing during more than seven years of clinical experience and nine years as a teacher.

Caroline has complete responsibility for the ENB Infectious Diseases Nursing Course and more recently the ENB Tuberculosis Care Course (for nurses and allied professionals).

Lovelle Smith, RGN, ENB 276, 934

Lovelle is currently a senior staff nurse at the John Hunter Clinic, HIV/GUM Directorate, the Chelsea and Westminster NHS Trust, London. She has a particular interest in black women's sexual health issues.

Anita Weston

Anita is the Associate Dean in the School of Health, Community and Social Policy at the Wolfson Institute of Health Science at Thames Valley University, London, and editor of Barrier Protection Digest.

For the past seven years she has been programme leader for the ENB 275/6 course, first at Riverside College of Health Studies, then at Thames Valley University. Anita has an international reputation as an expert in her field, having co-led HIV/AIDS nursing courses in India, and she has published material commissioned for the World Health Organisation and the Health Education Authority, as well as the nursing press.

Tracy Wright, RGN and DipHE in Professional Nursing

Tracy has worked in a sexual health clinic in East Berkshire for five years. During that time she has gained qualifications and experience in GU medicine (ENB 276), family planning (ENB 901), HIV and AIDS and teaching.

She has recently gained promotion to Sister and will be working in a GU clinic in West Berkshire.

Foreword

In 1991, myself and colleagues at the Riverside College of Health Studies set up the English National Board 275 Course in 'Caring for Persons with Sexually Transmitted Diseases', now called the ENB 276 Course 'Caring for Persons with Genito-Urinary Infections and Related Problems'. This course has run successfully since 1991, first at the Riverside College of Health Studies, London, and now at the Wolfson Institute of Health Sciences, Thames Valley University, London.

Students on the course are recruited mostly from a genito-urinary background and we have had students from the Hong Kong Department of Health and the British Army and Navy. During my long association with the course as Programme Leader, I have constantly been impressed by the level of commitment, motivation and genuine interest of the students, and by their shared desire to increase the profile of the care of the individuals with sexually transmitted infections (STIs), not only to the public whom we serve, but also to other health care professionals.

With this in mind, I was delighted when approached by the Nursing Times in 1997 to co-ordinate a series of articles on STIs. Most of these were written by past students of the ENB 276 course. The first series was so successful that a second series was commissioned in 1998.

This book is an up-to-date collection of those articles, most of which have been now extended and updated. As well as past students, other contributors include health advisers, clinical staff and nurse teachers. A chapter on psychosexual issues has been added to help give an overall perspective on the care of people with these infections.

While the numbers of new cases of STIs continues to rise in the United Kingdom, especially cases of chlamydia, genital warts and genital herpes, STIs can be said to be a major public health concern. Therefore we, as health care professionals, should be kept informed about them in order that we may offer our patients accurate and helpful care and advice, in whichever health care setting we find ourselves.

It is with great pride that I, on behalf of all the contributing authors, present this collection to you and hope that it goes some way to helping improve the care of those people with STIs with whom we come into contact as health care professionals.

Anita Weston

February 1999

1. Casting a long shadow – the sexually transmitted disease in history

Marsh Gelbart

NEW ILLNESS, OLD ATTITUDES

Human history has been shaped by disease to a greater extent than is commonly appreciated. Human behaviour has, in turn, influenced the incidence, prevalence and pathogenesis of various diseases.

Of all the contagious illnesses, perhaps none are as closely interrelated with human activities and attitudes as the sexually transmitted infections (STIs). Disruption caused by war, pressure from population growth and urbanisation have all played their part in creating the preconditions for epidemics. In addition, trade, colonisation and travel have led to contact between cultures with limited resistance to each other's communicable illnesses.

Sexually transmitted diseases have a long pedigree. They are mentioned in the Bible and in ancient Chinese and Greek medical texts. Up until the 15th century the most common STI is thought to have been gonorrhoea which, untreated, can lead to infertility and various chronic conditions. However, gonorrhoea is generally not life threatening.

In the 15th century a new, deadly, sexually transmitted pestilence took Europe by storm. Syphilis, or the 'Great Pox' as it was known, reached pandemic proportions. Millions of Europeans succumbed to the effects of *Treponema pallidum*, the organism responsible for syphilis. From contemporary descriptions, it seems that syphilis was more virulent than the disease we know today. Its pustular lesions were seen as a symbol of licentiousness and shame. Like most STIs, syphilis had social and political ramifications beyond the strict bounds of medicine. Countries wasted little time in blaming the illness on their political rivals: to the English it was the French Disease; for the Italians it became known as the Spanish Complaint.

From where did syphilis emerge? One possibility is that the disease arrived as a result of transoceanic exchange. This concept, developed by the historian William H. McNeill, states that when societies come into contact for the first time, they lack natural resistance to each other's infections (McNeill, 1979). Syphilis is thought to have been brought back to Europe after Columbus and his sailors discovered the New World of the Americas in 1492, before which the disease was unknown in Europe. In return they left behind devastating diseases, such as measles and smallpox, to which the Amerindians had no natural immunity. Transoceanic exchange is a powerful tool, and one which helps explain the epidemiology of many diseases and, at first glance, would explain the advent of syphilis in Europe. In 1494 Charles VIII of France invaded Naples with a mercenary army made up of men from all over Europe. Among their ranks will have been Spanish soldiers who had returned from the Americas infected with syphilis. By the time the Naples war was over, syphilis would have spread, via brothels, throughout the army. Soldiers then took syphilis back to their countries of origin, starting a European pandemic.

However, there is a school of thought which suggests that the Columbus/syphilis equation does not add up (Luger, 1993). Only a handful of Spanish soldiers who had accompanied Columbus went on to besiege Naples. The tight time-scale between returning from the voyage and the conclusion of the siege also undermines the case for syphilis originating in the Americas. Even given the traditional licentiousness of men at war, it does seem unlikely that the Spanish mercenaries were to blame. Pandemics breed moral panic; it was thought that syphilis was a punishment from God. People often look for a source of their suffering – someone or something to blame. The Spanish explorers and the American continent seemed to fit the bill in the case of syphilis.

Another possibility is that syphilis was not a new illness, but an old one in a new guise. Yaws, caused by a spirochaete seemingly identical to syphilis, had been endemic in Europe for centuries. It caused localised ulcers and open sores, usually on the lower limbs. Traditionally transmitted by skin-to-skin contact, classically between children sharing a bed, yaws coexisted with its host population in a delicate ecological balance. Europe in the 15th century was in transition, held in the grip of war and torn by social upheaval. These conditions broke down and established sexual taboos and restraints. The balance was disturbed, and the spirochaete exploited a new avenue of transmission: sexual contact. Population growth and urbanisation may also have accelerated the dissemination of STIs. Some historians have argued that populations must reach a certain critical mass before disease outbreaks occur. Certainly the squalor and close proximity endured by the majority of urban populations present a breeding ground for disease of all kinds. The role of cities in breaking sexual prohibitions has been unprecedented: 'Certainly people had sex regardless of where they lived, but cities created options. The sheer density of *Homo sapiens* populations, coupled with the anonymity of urban life, guaranteed greater sexual activity and experimentation' (Garrett, 1994).

SYMPTOMS AND ATTITUDES

After an initial period – probably of several decades – syphilis declined in virulence as the target population became accommodated to it. Yet it remained a scourge from 1495 right through to the 1940s. It was particularly feared thanks to its visible stigmata and the fact that the disease could be passed vertically to offspring. Syphilis caused a bewildering sequence of symptoms, ranging from disfiguring lesions to insidious nerve damage and mental disorientation. Medical techniques to combat syphilis were ineffectual. For centuries, treatment options were based on mercury ointments; in the 19th century the favoured options were crude preparations based on arsenic. All were painful and toxic.

Traditionally, hospitals were reluctant to accept patients suffering from venereal disease and specialist hospitals became necessary. The first of these was established in Russia by Catherine the Great in 1770. Incidentally, Catherine, despite folklore to the contrary, did not suffer from syphilis – unlike other historical worthies such as Henry VIII, and a string of 15th- and 16th-century popes (Morton, 1991). Other major European countries followed suit in establishing specialist hospitals for venereal diseases. In Britain these were known as lock hospitals. The term lock was a corruption of the mediaeval word loque. A loque was a communal rag with which lepers had to wipe clean their sores before being allowed to enter the isolation houses set aside for them.

The disapproval with which various societies looked upon those suffering from STIs was a hindrance to their treatment and prevention: 'There was not only a public health problem. There was also a social or attitudinal problem. In mid-19th-century UK 'VD' was seen as unmentionable, sinful and degrading. In a man such an infection was a tragedy or a sign of depravity. In a woman it was a crime' (Hansdfield and Hoel, 1997).

Given the prevailing social attitudes, it is no surprise to find restrictive legislation being used to mitigate the effects of STIs. The legislation enacted tended to do more harm than good. The classic British example is the Contagious Diseases Act of 1864. This allowed the compulsory arrest, examination and treatment of women considered, by an all-male board, to be of loose morals. Women were detained in the so-called canary wards, their identity made clear by the bright yellow garments they were forced to wear. The combination of poor diagnostic techniques – the organism that caused gonorrhoea was not identified until 1879 – and the often toxic 'cures' inflicted upon these poor women, makes the modern-day reader cringe. Treatment of syphilis remained largely ineffective until the 1907 discovery by Paul Erlich of salvarsan, medicine's original 'magic bullet'.

The next breakthrough in the control of STIs came about during the First World War. As is always the case in human history, war and dislocation led to an increase in STIs. Worried by the high rate of STIs in the armed forces, the British government of the day was forced to act. In the UK, the Public Health (Venereal Diseases) Regulations of 1916 introduced free and confidential treatment for STIs. Attendance at the new clinics which sprang up around the country was voluntary. People could attend without fear of stigma.

After the war, some other industrial countries were slow to adopt Britain's path. The USA in particular continued to have a problem with STIs. In the 1920s, on average, almost half a million Americans contracted syphilis each year, and close to 700,000 contracted gonorrhoea (Handsfield and Hoel, 1997). Prevailing harsh social attitudes against STIs proved ineffective in controlling their spread.

The Second World War also saw a massive increase in STIs world-wide, and a consequent increase in the efforts to control them. This time there was a genuine breakthrough in the treatment of disease which came about through the introduction of penicillin. Penicillin was used on a large scale, despite residual moral scruples, to treat the many thousands of soldiers who had contracted syphilis.

MEDICINE, MORALITY AND MORTALITY

After the war the struggle against STIs appeared to have been won: the 'Great Pox' had been largely defeated in the developed world. Effective treatment was available and, in the UK at least, it was confidential and free at source. This encouraged greater sexual freedom.

From the 1960s onwards, availability of the oral contraceptive pill led to a reduction in use of barrier methods of contraception, thus increasing the chances of disease transmission. From the 1950s the incidence of STI cases, both nationally and internationally, showed an increase. Gonorrhoea rates in the 1960s and 1970s mirrored the increased level of casual sex. In England and Wales in 1971, 57,571 people were diagnosed as having gonorrhoea (Morton, 1995). In the USA in the early 1980s, 2.5 million people were catching gonorrhoea annually, and it was becoming increasingly resistant to standard treatments (Garrett, 1994).

Perhaps more disturbingly, there was a notable increase in the incidence of a new wave of STIs: genital warts, genital herpes, non-specific urethritis, and chlamydia. From the 1970s, in urban centres in the western industrialised countries, there was an even more precipitous rise in STIs amongst gay men than in the population as a whole (Garrett, 1994).

Then came HIV (human immunodeficiency virus). For the first time since the 15th century populations were, and still are, confronted by a life-threatening pandemic, primarily spread through sexual contact. In the West the majority of the initial target populations for HIV were on the fringes of society: gay men, intravenous drug users, and refugees from impoverished Haiti. HIV came as a shock to societies who thought they had conquered the scourge of pestilence. The growth of industrialised civilisation and technologically sophisticated medicine hadn't prevented old patterns of social behaviour reasserting themselves.

Plague – of any kind – leads to panic and resultant prejudice. As mentioned earlier, when faced with infectious disease, people search for scapegoats. In the case of an illness which involved sexual transmission, the temptation to brand the initial target populations as pariahs was intense. Sex, morality and mortality provide a potent combination. When the extent of the HIV epidemic in Africa – which primarily affects heterosexuals – became evident, a similar unpleasant current of prejudice emerged against black Africans.

Medical science has worked frantically to develop a remedy for HIV. Despite the success of triple combination therapies in slowing down the disease process, no cure is in sight. Additionally, combination therapies are too expensive for all but the most wealthy societies. Health care and public utilities in the developing countries are desperately over-stretched. It has been said that if the cure for HIV was one glass of pure, uncontaminated water, then that would be beyond the means of much of Africa's population (Zarembo, 1997). In November 1997 the World Health Organisation (WHO) estimated that 30.6 million people were living with HIV, the vast majority in developing countries (Lichfield, 1997). In Africa the situation is catastrophic – over 20 million people are thought to have HIV. By the year 2001 a similar figure is expected to exist in India, where the fight against HIV transmission has been hampered by complacency and ignorance (Popham, 1998). The only viable hope for the millions of people in the developing world who already have HIV, and for the greater number at risk, is the development of a vaccine. In the interim, health education and the encouragement of condom use remain the most effective options.

Health care programmes to limit the spread of STIs are vital, not only to combat the sequelae of illnesses such as gonorrhoea and syphilis, but also because they, along with other STIs, facilitate the transmission of HIV. The scale of the problem should not be underestimated. The WHO estimated that in 1995 there were 12 million new cases of syphilis amongst adults world-wide. In the same year there were an estimated 62 million cases of gonorrhoea.

Modelling techniques used by the WHO and posted on their Internet site suggest that, 'by curing or preventing one hundred cases of syphilis among an STI high-risk (core) group, approximately 1,200 HIV infections linked to those one hundred episodes of syphilis could be prevented over the coming 10-year period'. Unlike the civilisation of the 15th century, we have a scientific understanding of the modes of transmission of STIs. We can limit the devastation of this new 'Great Pox' by modifying our sexual behaviour. If resources are released grudgingly, if societies are unable to discuss sexuality openly, or if people with HIV are stigmatised, then the task will be impossible.

References

Garrett, Laurie (1994) *The coming plague*. London: Penguin Books.

Hansdfield, H. and Hoel, D. (1997) Sex, Science and Society. *Postgraduate Medicine*; 101: 5, 268–278.

Lichfield, John (1997) Lethal epidemic is much larger than feared. *The Independent*; Friday 27th November, p.7.

Luger, Anton (1993) The origins of syphilis. Clinical and epidemiologic considerations of the Columbian theory. *Sexually Transmitted Diseases*; 20: 2, 110–117.

McNeill, William H. (1979) *Plagues and peoples*. London: Penguin Books.

Morton, Robert (1995) The development of genito-urinary medicine services. *British Journal of Sexual Medicine*; January/February, 20–22.

Morton, Robert (1991) Did Catherine the Great of Russia have syphilis? *Genito-urinary Medicine*; 498–502.

Popham, Peter (1998) Fear grips India as AIDS epidemic looms closer. *The Irish Independent*; Saturday 2nd May 1998.

Zarembo, Alan (1997) Hope and despair. *Newsweek*; Monday 8th December, pp 40–47.

2. Epidemiology

Anita Weston

INTRODUCTION

In our world of fewer than six billion people, more and more men, women and children are becoming infected with sexually transmitted infections (STIs) each year. In 1995 alarm bells were sounded when the World Health Organisation (WHO) estimated that over a third of a billion new sexually transmitted infections would occur in that year alone (WHO, 1995). As this report only focused on those infections which were potentially curable, it clearly underestimated the real size of an evolving pandemic of STIs that continues to expand as we come to the end of the 20th century.

Every STI could potentially be a new HIV (human immunodeficiency virus) infection, as STIs are an indication that unprotected sex has taken place. The presence of inflammation or genital lesions greatly increases the risk of sexual transmission of HIV; therefore, increasing numbers of STIs are fuelling the spread of HIV.

STIs may cause infertility in both men and women. They cause many serious complications in women, such as pelvic inflammatory disease (PID) and ectopic pregnancy. Many STIs can be passed on to infants during pregnancy and childbirth. Their effects include abortion and stillbirth of the foetus; eye infections and pneumonia in the newborn child (WHO, 1995). Treating such complications may be costly, and is unaffordable in many parts of the world. Also, the psychological impact of STIs may be profound on the individual and on his or her current and future sexual relationships.

FACING THE FACTS

In the United Kingdom the number of new cases of STIs continues to rise, especially chlamydia, genital herpes and genital warts (Fig 1), with total diagnoses of acute STIs rising by 7% between 1995 and 1996 (PHLS, 1998). Increased numbers of diagnoses were associated particularly with teenage cases, which would indicate that this is a group which needs to be continually considered and targeted with sexual health promotion initia-

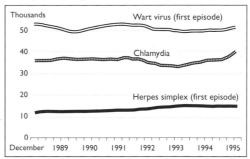

Fig 1 New cases of selected conditions in England

tives. The Durex Report of 1998 (London International Group, 1998), a summary of consumer research into the sexual attitudes and behaviour of 10,000 respondents in the British population, notes the degree of ignorance among sexually active teenagers, and finds this both surprising and worrying, considering the amount of information freely available to them.

The findings of the Durex Global Sex Survey of 1997 suggested that the practice of safer sex was being forgotten (London International Group, 1997). The survey found that people were having more sex than ever before, with the French being the most sexually active, having an average of 151 episodes of sexual intercourse per year. The British figure was 113 times per year. The survey found that those interviewed believed sexual satisfaction to be more important than concerns over STIs, HIV or unwanted pregnancy, and concluded by advocating the need to intensify safer sex education globally. Only 25% of the British respondents said they put great importance, during sexual intercourse, on not contacting or spreading HIV, and just 3% said they were concerned about other STIs.

Finally, the survey called for a greater responsibility from the medical and nursing professions for sex education as, of the 10,000 adults questioned in 14 countries, only 2% cited doctors and nurses as a source of information.

THE HIDDEN PROBLEM

Clarke carried out an international study in 1995 to explore awareness of STIs (Clarke, 1995). Only 1% of the 959 UK citizens interviewed had heard of chlamydia and 2% had heard of genital warts. Considering that these two infections are the most common STIs in the UK, this finding is very worrying and suggests that public health promotion campaigns targeting STIs should become a government priority.

The continual rise in the number of cases of STIs has promoted debate about the failure of the targets for sexual health set out by the *Health of the Nation* White Paper in July 1992 (Adler, 1997). One of the targets was to reduce the incidence of STIs, with a particular emphasis on gonorrhoea. Although the number of cases of gonorrhoea did decline between 1992 and 1994, thereafter there has been a gradual increase in the number of cases being seen in genito-urinary medicine (GUM) clinics. There was an increase of 5% in 1995 (12,359 cases) over 1994 (DoH, 1996), and there were 20% more diagnoses of gonorrhoea in 1996 than in 1995 (PHLS, 1998).

Recent newspaper reports suggest that Britain is facing a new epidemic of herpes simplex virus (HSV), as reported by the GUM clinics (Austin, 1997). Government statistics allegedly reveal an increase in the incidence of genital herpes of 50% between 1987 and 1997, with more than 27,500 cases reported in 1997. Research has shown that one in five of the population could be infected by the incurable virus (Adler, 1997).

The infection *Chlamydia trachomatis* is the most common bacterial STI seen in this country. It causes non-specific urethritis in men and, if left untreated, may cause epididymitis and infertility. Chlamydia infects the female cervix and may go unnoticed by an infected woman as there are often no symptoms. However, if left untreated chlamydia can lead to PID and infertility. Many cases of infertility can be traced back to infection with chlamydia.

It is precisely because infections such as chlamydia and gonorrhoea can be hidden, in women especially, that a sexual health check-up at a GUM clinic is recommended if there is a change of sexual partner or there is a non-monogamous relationship. Under such circumstances, the same recommendation should be made for men, although if they have a bacterial STI they usually display more obvious symptoms.

PROMOTING SEXUAL HEALTH

An effective sexual health promotion strategy which the British could learn from is that of The National Institute of Public Health in Stockholm, Sweden, responsible for co-ordinating STI and HIV prevention in Sweden (Folkhalsointitutet, 1995). It achieves this by promoting safer sexual behaviour, counteracting fear and anxiety and alleviating the personal and social consequences of HIV and STIs. The Institute works closely with central and local government agencies and the community, and maintains international links with the United Nations and European Union AIDS programme.

It is well known that the Swedes have a more liberal attitude towards sex and sex education than we do in Britain. The Institute's policy is that sexual activity is an important component of life and therefore it inculcates a positive view of sex and personal relations, the implication being that people can enjoy life in spite of the risks that HIV and STIs pose. The Swedes believe that knowledge of these infections and how they are transmitted can help considerably in allaying the apprehension many people feel about discussing them.

Through systematic preventive measures, including national publicity campaigns and media coverage giving factual and safer sex information, the Swedes have successfully reduced the frequency of many STIs, such as gonorrhoea and syphilis, and they are currently targeting the problem of chlamydia using a similar strategy. Clarke's study (Clarke, 1995) found that 55% of Swedes had heard of chlamydia, compared to the paltry 1% of British citizens. This study is proof in itself that mass media public awareness campaigns do work, as we witnessed in this country in the late 1980s with the government's HIV and AIDS awareness campaign.

The incidence of STIs will continue to increase unabated while people remain ignorant of the facts. This ignorance is not confined to the general public – many health care workers are often ill-informed and in the dark when it comes to advising clients about STIs. Knowledge of STIs should not just be the province of a relatively small number of specialist nurses, but should be of interest to all nurses and health care providers, whether they work in hospital, in general practice or in the community. We must keep ourselves informed about these infections in order that we can offer our clients accurate and helpful advice and optimum sexual health care.

References

Adler, M.W. (1997) Sexual health: a health of the nation failure. *British Medical Journal*; 314: 7096, 1743–1747.

Austin, M. Herpes epidemic feared as new cases reach high. *The Sunday Times*; 2 November 1997, p.13.

Clarke, P. (1995) *Awareness of sexually transmitted diseases – an international study*. New Orleans, Louisiana, USA: International Society for Sexually Transmitted Diseases Research.

Department of Health (1996) *Statistical Bulletin: Sexually Transmitted Diseases, England 1995*; Bulletin 1996/14. London: DoH.

Durex Global Sex Survey 1997. London: London International Group.

The Durex Report 1998: A summary of consumer research into sexual attitudes and behaviour. London: London International Group.

Public Health Laboratory Service (PHLS), Communicable Disease Report Supplement (1998) *New cases seen at genito-urinary medicine clinics, England 1996*; 8: 1. London: PHLS.

The National Institute of Public Health (Folkhalsointitutet) (1995) *STD and HIV Prevention in Sweden*. Stockholm, Sweden.

World Health Organisation (WHO) (1995) *Sexually transmitted disease – three hundred and thirty-three million new curable cases in 1995*; press release WHO/64. Geneva: WHO.

3. Striking back at syphilis

Anita Weston

INTRODUCTION

Syphilis is not a common sexually transmitted infection (STI) in the United Kingdom. The number of new cases of infections of syphilis reported each year has fallen consistently since the 1930s (Fig 1) (Public Health Laboratory Service, 1997). However, this trend should not lead us into complacency, as the World Health Organisation (WHO) estimates that there are 12 million new cases of infections of syphilis world-wide each year, with the largest numbers of cases being found in southern and

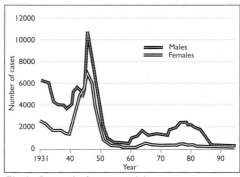

Fig 1 Cases of infectious syphilis

south-east Asia and sub-Saharan Africa (Sherrand et al, 1997). Also, the re-emergence of syphilis as a significant public health problem in the USA (United States Public Health Service, 1996) and Russia, the Baltic States and Poland (Linglöf, 1995), has begun to have a direct impact on the number of new cases of infections of syphilis being seen in the UK (Linglöf, 1995; Deayton et al, 1997).

The government statistical service, in its summary of information recorded by NHS genito-urinary medicine (GUM) clinics in 1995, reported that the number of new cases of infectious syphilis in the UK in 1995 was 283, a fall of 7% from 1993 (DoH, 1996). Males accounted for 66% of new infections. New cases of non-infectious syphilis rose by 4% to 1,134 cases. The total of 1,417 cases remained at the continuing low level recorded since the late 1980s. The summary noted that an estimated 32% of cases of infections of syphilis in males were reported as being acquired by men who have sex with men. It should be noted here that, contrary to the UK trend, in Bristol between January and December 1997 there were 42 cases of infectious syphilis (Battu et al, 1997) compared with only two cases in the preceding three years (PHLS, 1997).

SYMPTOMS

Syphilis is a bacterial infection caused by the spirochaete *Treponema pallidum*. This tiny spiral-shaped micro-organism was first discovered by Schaudinn and Hoffman in 1905. It is one of the pathogenic treponemes that infect humans, and can be found in serum from a primary or secondary syphilitic lesion using a microscope with a dark-ground condenser.

Treponema pallidum is mainly transmitted through sexual contact. The micro-organisms gain access at the site of inoculation, usually the genitalia, and produce the primary lesion, known as a chancre. The micro-organisms are then disseminated from the site of inoculation throughout many organs in the body. An immune response develops, serological tests for syphilis (STS) become positive and the primary infection heals, but thereafter, the disease becomes a chronic inflammatory condition affecting many organs.

The course of the disease is usually divided into four stages:

- primary syphilis;
- secondary syphilis;
- latent syphilis;
- tertiary syphilis.

Infectious or early syphilis may include the primary, secondary and early latent stages if mucosal ulcerative manifestations are present. If left untreated the disease progresses to the latent stage and may then develop into tertiary syphilis, which is characterised by neurosyphilis or cardiovascular (gummatous) syphilis.

DIAGNOSIS

A sexual history should be taken, and as much of today's syphilis is acquired abroad, a travel history may also be relevant. A full physical examination of the patient, checking for skin rashes or any genital ulcers should be carried out. All genital ulcers should have a serum sample taken from them and this should be prepared for dark-ground microscopy. A blood sample should also be taken for serological testing to detect antibodies.

Serological testing for syphilis (STS)

A venereal disease research laboratory (VDRL) test identifies non-specific non-treponemal antibodies and will identify disease and disease activity.

A fluorescent treponemal antibody absorption test (FTA-ABS) identifies specific treponemal antibodies and confirms the probability of past or present treponemal infection. A *Treponema pallidum* haemagglutination (TPHA) test can be carried out – this is similar to the FTA-ABS test but identifies the antigen.

Primary syphilis

A primary chancre begins as a small red macule that enlarges and develops through a papular stage, becoming eroded to form a round, indurated painless ulcer. If untreated this ulcer usually heals after four to eight weeks. The chancre appears in the skin or mucosa, at the site of entry of the organism, between one and twelve weeks after exposure to the infection. The site of entry is usually the vulva, cervix or penis, but depending on the sexual practice engaged in, the chancre could appear in the rectum, on the lips or in the mouth. There is a heavy concentration of chronic inflammatory cells, particularly lymphocytes and plasma cells. The chancre ulcerates and there may be painless enlargement of local lymph nodes. The chancre is highly infectious, with many spirochaetes present within it. At this stage the spirochaetes have already migrated throughout the body. Depending on the site of the chancre, the patient may not notice it as it is painless.

Secondary syphilis

Secondary syphilis typically occurs one to three months after the initial infection and is characterised by the following features:

- mild fever or flu-like symptoms with anorexia and a sore throat;
- malaise;
- lymphadenopathy;
- patchy hair loss;
- a variety of skin rashes, often concentrated on the body trunk, the palms of the hands and the soles of the feet.

In addition, there may be mucosal involvement, such as shallow ulcers in the genital mucosa and the formation of warty growths around the genitalia, called *Condylomata lata*. Such manifestations can be infectious as the micro-organism is very active at this time.

Latent syphilis

If untreated the infected person passes into the latent stage about two years after initially acquiring syphilis. The person will be asymptomatic but will still harbour the infection although, at this stage, will no longer be sexually infectious. However, it is important to note that at all stages of syphilis, mother to foetus transfer can occur.

During the latent stages, symptoms of secondary syphilis may recur.

Tertiary syphilis

Tertiary syphilis occurs after a period of latency that can be between 3 and 30 years. It affects about one-third of people who have untreated syphilis. There are two main patterns of disease:

- The blood vessels become damaged and there is a poor blood supply to the tissues. The result of this may be a thoracic aortic aneurysm.

▶ Areas of necrosis known as 'gummas' may develop in several tissues, including the bones.

The tissues most commonly involved by the disease progression are the skin, mucous membranes, subcutaneous and submucous tissues, bones, joints and ligaments. However, there may also be more serious systemic effects.

Table I Systemic effects of tertiary syphilis

Cardiovascular system (cardiovascular syphilis)
Aortic aneurysm formation, widening of aortic valve ring producing incompetence.

Liver
Gummas may develop and resolve to scars.

Central nervous system (neurosyphilis)
▶ Meningovascular disease: ischaemic lesions, cranial nerve damage, strokes, sensory abnormalities.
▶ Parenchynal disease: infection with spirochaetes causes dementia; also known as general paralysis of the insane (GPI).
▶ *Tabes dorsalis.*
▶ Loss of spinal posterior columns leading to sensory loss.

Eyes
Argyll Robertson pupils that accommodate but do not react to light – may be seen in neurosyphilis.

Testes
Gummas produce firm swellings, simulating tumours.

Bones
Gummas produce areas of bone necrosis; hard palate may be perforated.

Due to curative treatment and the widespread use of antibiotics, tertiary syphilis is rare in the UK today, but it is sometimes found, particularly in the elderly, and may be misdiagnosed (Bremner & Radcliffe, 1993). Therefore, doctors and nurses should familiarise themselves with the symptoms of tertiary syphilis, especially when caring for elderly people who are diagnosed with dementia-related illnesses.

TREATMENT

Standard treatment for primary syphilis is procaine penicillin: 600,000 international units (IUs) daily, intramuscularly, for 10 to 12 days. If the patient is allergic to penicillin, 2–3g of oxytetracycline or erythromycin can be given daily in divided doses for 10–12 days. The patient should refrain from sexual intercourse until all lesions have healed and follow-up serological tests show that the infection has been successfully treated. This takes about three months, but intercourse using a condom could be practised during this time.

Ninety-five per cent of patients will be cured using this regime; the remaining 5% may have to be re-treated. It is possible to treat all stages of syphilis with varying regimes, but some organ damage caused by tertiary syphilis will be irreversible.

Jarisch Herzheimer reaction

It is important that before treating the patient, he is warned of the possibility of a Jarisch Herzheimer reaction. This reaction may occur a few hours after therapy, and occasionally immediately after. Symptoms are fever, tachycardia and a widespread rash, which usually last for a few hours. The patient should be advised to rest in bed, take plenty of fluids and an antipyretic.

Follow-up

The patient should be seen as follows:

- monthly for three months following treatment;
- three-monthly up to one year after the start of treatment;
- at two years after the start of the treatment.

At each visit, the patient should be clinically examined and have bloods taken for VDRL and TPHA. Relapse with the infection is possible.

Screening

Screening for syphilis using serological testing is carried out routinely in the UK in all pregnant women attending antenatal clinics, in all patients who attend genito-urinary medicine clinics for a sexual health screen, in all people donating blood, and often in elderly and mental health patients. As a result of such screening a reasonable idea of the prevalence of syphilis in the UK can be obtained.

Congenital syphilis is now rare in the UK. Penicillin is effective in preventing a mother passing syphilis to her infant if given within the first six months of pregnancy.

Partner notification

Partner notification is an important aspect of the management of any patient presenting with syphilis, or indeed any other STI. In GUM clinics, the health adviser has a crucial role in assisting with partner notification. This may be done informally, by helping patients to find appropriate ways of raising the subject of their infection with their partner(s), discussing safer sex and suggesting that they visit the clinic themselves for a sexual health check-up. Health advisers can also give the patient a 'contact slip' to give or send to a partner, or this can be sent anonymously by the clinic. The contact slip explains that the partner may have been exposed to an STI, and suggests they make an appointment for a check-up with the clinic. The identity of the index case patient is not disclosed using this method.

Conclusion

Although syphilis is often viewed as one of yesterday's diseases, it certainly has not gone away. Thanks to a widespread screening programme in the UK, and the easy availability of treatment, we have been able to control the problem and very rarely experience patients with tertiary syphilis or who die with the manifestations of this often debilitating stage of the disease. However, we need to be alert to the fact that syphilis is on the increase in many parts of the world and that we are therefore likely to see more and more cases of 'imported' syphilis, both in Britons who travel abroad and in foreign visitors or immigrants to Britain.

Case study

Mark, a 42-year-old single businessman attended his local GUM clinic with a small round indurated ulcer on the shaft of his penis. His sexual and travel history showed that he had a regular girlfriend of five months duration who used the oral contraceptive pill. He had last had unprotected sex with his girlfriend one month ago. However, three weeks ago he had attended a conference in Kiev, in the Ukraine, and had drunk a lot of vodka with his colleagues and had unprotected sex with a young woman he met in a bar there. He returned to England and, nine days later, noticed the sore on the shaft of his penis. Mark was confused by this as it didn't hurt. At first he thought it could be herpes. Luckily, his girlfriend was away when he returned to England and he had not yet had sex with her since his travels. Mark appeared rather anxious and embarrassed.

On clinical examination, the sore had the appearance of a primary syphilitic chancre. Dark-ground microscopy revealed the presence of spirochaetes in serum taken from the chancre. A blood sample was taken for VDRL, FTA–ABS and TPHA testing. Mark was given a diagnosis of primary syphilis. The nurse asked Mark if he knew anything about syphilis. He said 'not really', so she gave a brief explanation of the infection. The nurse explained to Mark that it was advisable to refrain from sexual intercourse until his chancre had healed and treatment was completed, then he could resume using condoms. The nurse asked Mark if he had had sex with anyone since returning from Kiev, but he said he had not. As his regular girlfriend was going to be away for another month herself, Mark felt he didn't want her to know about his diagnosis.

This was his decision and the nurse respected this, but advised use of condoms with his girlfriend when she returned. Mark said this could be difficult as his girlfriend was on the pill and she would wonder why he suddenly wanted to use condoms, but he said he would find a way around it. The nurse asked Mark if he had any questions, and told him that he could call her at the clinic at any time if there was anything else he wanted to know about his diagnosis. An information leaflet about syphilis was given to Mark to read in his own time. The doctor prescribed a ten day course of procaine penicillin, 600,000 IUs to be given intra-muscularly daily. Mark was warned about the possibility of the Jarisch Herzheimer reaction and was then given his first injection. Mark was given an appointment time to return the following day for his second injection. He left the clinic calmly, saying he was glad he had found out what was wrong with him and that it was treatable.

References

Battu, V.R., Horner, P.J., Taylor, P.K., Jephcott, A.E. et al (1997) Locally acquired heterosexual outbreak of syphilis in Bristol. *The Lancet;* 350: 9084, 1100–1101.

Bremner, A. and Radcliffe, K. (1993) Missing the diagnosis of neurosyphilis. *Journal of Sexual Medicine;* May/June, p.14.

Deayton, J., French, P. and Nicoll, A. (1997) *Syphilis in the UK – impact of the epidemic in the former Soviet Union.* Oxford: MSSVD.

Department of Health (1996) *Statistical Bulletin: Sexually Transmitted Diseases, England 1995;* Bulletin 1996/14. London: DoH.

Linglöf, T. (1995) Rapid increase of syphilis and gonorrhoea in parts of the former USSR. *Sexually Transmitted Diseases;* 22: 160–161.

Public Health Laboratory Service (PHLS) (1997) An outbreak of infectious syphilis in Bristol. Communicable Disease Report; 7: 33, 291. London: PHLS.

Public Health Laboratory Service (PHLS) (1997) Sexually transmitted diseases quarterly; Syphilis in England and Wales. *Communicable Diseases Report;* 7: 22, 192, London: PHSL.

Sherrand, J., Luzzi, G. Edwards, A. (1997) Imported syphilis and other sexually transmitted infections among UK travellers to Russia and Poland. *Genito-urinary Medicine;* 73: 1, 75.

United States Public Health Service (1996) *Sexually Transmitted Disease Surveillance 1995.* Atlanta: Centers for Disease Control and Prevention.

4. Gonorrhoea: symptoms and treatment

Heledd Nicholas and Anita Weston

INTRODUCTION

Gonorrhoea, despite the *Health of the Nation* initiative, has not gone away. It is a universally common, highly contagious bacterial infection affecting columnar or transitional epithelium. It can be found in the urethra or rectum in males, in the urethra, cervical canal or rectum in women, and in the pharynx, tonsils and conjunctival sac in both sexes (the last, especially in the newborn). It can spread from tissue to tissue.

Unlike other serious sexually transmissible infections (STIs), such as syphilis or HIV infection, it has a relatively short incubation period. In some cases, symptoms such as a discharge or dysuria can be seen 24 hours after infection. It is highly infectious – there is a two in three chance of a woman catching it from a single sexual encounter with an infected person. For men, the risk is one in three.

Its incidence is increasing. The World Health Organisation estimates that worldwide there are around 40 million new cases each year. Some unofficial estimates put the figure for new cases as high as 200 million (Bingham, 1995a). Although the number of cases in Western countries has steadily decreased – some, such as Sweden, have almost eliminated the disease – the picture worldwide is mixed and changing (Bingham, 1995b).

After years of steady fall, in part prompted by the onset of AIDS in the 1980s and in part by better health education, contact tracing and treatment, gonorrhoea is now on the increase again in the UK and the USA. Figures for 1996 show that the number of patients with uncomplicated gonorrhoea has increased by almost one-sixth for men and one-seventh for women, compared with 1995 figures. This is a rise of almost 50% since the end of 1993. Roughly 8000 men and 4000 women who contacted gonorrhoea were seen at sexual health clinics that same year (Communicable Disease Centre, 1997).

In the UK, gonorrhoea is most likely to be seen among people from ethnic minorities, homosexuals and younger women. The key risk indicators include living in an inner city, coming from a deprived background, being single, first having sex at an early age, and having a history of sexual infection.

Almost half of all diagnosed UK cases are found in London. A study in south London showed that the incidence of gonorrhoea was 12 times higher in young people from black ethnic groups than their white counterparts (Low et al, 1997). This trend has remained constant since the 1950s. In 1960 the British Cooperative Clinical Group noted that people from the Afro-Caribbean community accounted for a quarter of all cases of gonorrhoea (Low et al, 1997).

Young women aged 16–19 have a higher incidence of gonorrhoea than the national average. Teenage women are up to 15 times more likely than women over 30 to contract gonorrhoea (Communicable Disease Surveillance Centre, 1997).

CLINICAL FEATURES

Gonorrhoea has been known since the earliest times. Descriptions of it can be found in the Old Testament of the Bible and in the writings of a Chinese emperor dated 2600BC.

Treatment has been steadily improving, and for the past 50 years gonorrhoea has been curable. However, the organism that causes it, *Neisseria gonorrhoeae*, has fought back. Its clinical features have changed, with studies showing that its incubation period is lengthening and, generally, the symptoms are less severe or absent (Bingham, 1995).

The number of cases of gonorrhoea caused by antibiotic-resistant isolates continues to increase. Gonorrhoea has shown itself to be particularly resistant to penicillin, with the emergence and spread of penicillinase producing *Neisseria gonorrhoeae* (PPNG) in the 1970s (Bignell, 1996). as a result, fluoroquinolones are now commonly the first choice of treatment, especially for rectal and pharyngeal gonorrhoea. In addition to PPNG, there now exist other types of antimicrobial resistance to *Neisseria gonorrhoeae*. These are classified into plasmid-mediated and chromosomially mediated strains.

There are also growing fears that asymptomatic infection is on the increase, but the incidence is, as yet, unproven. Although signs of infection can frequently be seen within a day, there are many instances where few or no symptoms are visible. Gonorrhoea in women and homosexual men usually has fewer or no symptoms, and a routine visual examination may reveal nothing.

Gonorrhoea is rarely life-threatening. However, in women, complications caused as a result of an infection rising through the genital tract can lead to pelvic inflammatory disease (PID), infertility, chronic pelvic pain and an increased risk of an ectopic pregnancy, *ophthalmia neonatorum* and premature delivery. More rarely, if the infection is left untreated, other complications such as arthritis and heart disease can occur as a result of disseminated gonococcal infection. In men, it can lead to urethral stricture, epididymitis, prostatitis and infertility.

Gonorrhoea factfile

Gonorrhoea infections in men outnumber those in women two to one, whereas for genito-urinary medicine cases generally the ratio is 0.9 to 1.[†]

- Almost half of all cases of gonorrhoea are diagnosed in London.
- Homosexual males make up 32% of cases in London, 19% outside the capital.
- People of Afro-Caribbean origin make up 53% of cases in large London centres and 43% in large provincial centres, whereas the figure is only 15% in small provincial clinics.
- Clinical microscopy can provide an immediate diagnosis and currently detects 89% of male urethral cases, but only 37% of female infections; fluoroquinolones have now overtaken penicillins as the treatment of choice in the UK.
- Patients report on average 1.5 contacts each, but overall only 0.5 contacts attend the clinics for examination. Within this figure, the rate attending large London clinics is half that attending small provincial clinics.

[†] *Source: Fitzgerald, M., Bedford, C. (1996) National Audit Development Project in Sexual Health*

DIAGNOSIS

Neisseria gonorrhoeae infects a wide range of mucosal surfaces, including the urethra, endocervix, fallopian tubes, genital glands (Bartholin's in women and Tyson's in men), prostate, testicles, rectum, pharynx and conjunctiva. It is highly infectious and is generally acquired through sexual contact. As mentioned earlier, the risk of acquiring it from a single sexual encounter with an infected person is 20–40% for men, and 60–90% for women. This difference arises because the vagina and cervix have a larger surface area within which to harbour infectious fluids than the male urethra.

The incubation period for gonorrhoea is usually two to five days, but it can be longer. In uncomplicated gonorrhoea men's symptoms are typically urethritis with a thick yellow-white discharge, and dysuria. One in ten men have no symptoms.

Women may have few or no symptoms and at examination everything may appear normal. Where symptoms are present these may include an increase in normal discharge, dysuria, dyspareunia, intermenstrual bleeding and lower abdominal pain. Cervicitis with an endocervical discharge may be seen on examination.

The majority of pharyngeal gonorrhoea is asymptomatic, with rates of infection being higher in homosexual men and heterosexual women than in heterosexual men. This is because the practice of fellatio presents more of a risk of oral infection with gonorrhoea than does the practice of cunnilingus (Edwards and Carne, 1998). The most common symptom is pharyngitis, causing a sore throat and very occasionally a purulent tonsillitis.

Because gonorrhoea and other STIs may be asymptomatic and may cause long-term morbidity it is important to take a detailed sexual history from the patient, to make a physical examination, and carry out microbiological tests. Resistant strains can be found globally, although some strains are more common in certain parts of the world. Therefore, it may be helpful to take a recent travel history from the patient at the time of sexual history taking.

Contact tracing is essential. Successful notification and treatment of sexual partners has been at the heart of Sweden's success story in curbing infection rates. This is particularly important given that two-thirds of men become reinfected (Daker-White et al, 1997).

Gonorrhoea is diagnosed by identifying Gram-negative intracellular diplococci on a Gram's stain smear or culture. This is normally around 95% sensitive. In men, samples are taken from the urethra, in women, the endocervix is the optimum site. However, gonorrhoea is isolated from the urethra in most cases and this should also be swabbed. Infection of the rectum occurs in around half of cases in women; it is rarely the only site of infection.

Where there is a history of anal sex, specimens should be taken from the rectum. People practising oral sex require throat swabs. Microscopy can provide an immediate diagnosis. However, this is not totally reliable, so cultures should also be taken.

The co-existence of other (STIs) with gonorrhoea is common, especially those of *Chlamydia trachomatis* and *Trichomonas vaginalis*. Co-infection with *Chlamydia trachomatis* is significant in both men and women and therefore combined antibiotic therapy at the time of the initial treatment for gonorrhoea may help reduce possible longer term complications, such as PID, ectopic pregnancy and infertility in women and epididymitis and infertility in men, which could occur as a result of untreated chlamydia.

As infection with gonorrhoea causes inflammation and a breakdown of mucosal surfaces, this provides a portal of entry for the human immunodeficiency virus (HIV). Therefore, being infected with gonorrhoea may considerably increase the individual's risk of being infected with HIV also.

TREATMENT

Treatment is usually a single dose of antibiotics (ciprofloxacin 250mg administrated immediately). Treatment may also be given to cover chlamydia infection (for example, doxycycline 200mg administered immediately, then 100mg once a day for ten days); specific treatment for pregnant women is also available (amoxycillin 3g administered immediately).

Early and appropriate action and avoidance of reinfection lessen the chance of complications. Contacts should also be seen, screened and treated. All patients should have follow-up screening two weeks later.

CONCLUSION

Treating the upsurge of gonorrhoea is crucial to tackling sexual health in the next millennium, and it is important that health care professionals are aware of the changing clinical presentation that we are now experiencing with gonorrhoea, especially as more and more cases appear to be asymptomatic in both men and women.

Case study

Jenny, 22, came to the sexual health clinic complaining of a slight itchy, white vaginal discharge which she had had on and off for six weeks. She had previously had vaginal thrush. Thinking this was the cause of the discharge, she had tried treating herself at home using vaginal pessaries bought from a chemist shop. These had not relieved the discomfort. She was not experiencing any other symptoms, such as dysuria or abdominal pain.

Jenny had a regular male partner, with whom she had been having a sexual relationship for the past four months. Their last sexual contact had been three days prior to her visit, when they had unprotected vaginal intercourse and oral sex. Condoms were their usual method of contraception, but they used them haphazardly. She had had one other male sexual partner in the previous eight months. Her present partner was aware of her visit to the clinic; he was asymptomatic.

A sexual health screening and examination was performed. A speculum was passed into the vagina to examine the cervix. Samples of discharge were taken using disposable plastic loops to test for *Trichomonas vaginalis*, *Candida albicans*, bacterial vaginosis, *Neisseria gonorrhoea* and *Chlamydia trachomatis*. The swabs for gonorrhoea were collected from the endocervix, urethra and pharynx for Gram's stain smear and culture.

The clinical examination of Jenny's vagina and cervix appeared normal. A bimanual examination did not show anything. The urinalysis and pregnancy test were negative. A sample of blood was taken to test for syphilis.

Examination of the slide under the microscope showed the presence of Gram-negative intracellular diplococci indicating gonorrhoea. Other tests were done on part of the sample, confirming the diagnosis.

Factors affecting the choice of drug treatment include the site of the infection, the strain of gonorrhoea, risk of pregnancy and, in global terms, where the patient had caught the disease, as there is a greater risk of resistance to antibiotics in some parts of the world. Patients should ideally be treated with a single dose of an antibiotic.

In Jenny's case, she was given a single 250mg dose of ciprofloxacin with epidemiological treatment for chlamydia. Epidemiological treatment is used in cases when the patient, while not having the disease, may be at risk of catching it. Gonorrhoea and chlamydia frequently go hand-in-hand. In Jenny's case, the treatment was 200mg of doxycycline on the first day, followed by a 100mg dose for nine days.

When Jenny was informed of the test results she was upset and shocked. Having a STI can induce a wide range of emotions in people, which can include anger, recrimination, shame, fear and confusion. It can threaten and damage relationships, so the practitioner needs to exercise skill and sensitivity when dealing with such issues.

Jenny was provided with information about gonorrhoea, including transmission, treatment and possible complications. She was advised on how to inform her current and past partners as she was worried about doing this. She was reassured about confidentiality, asked to reattend the clinic two weeks later and refrain from sex. Jenny was also provided with an explanatory leaflet and two contact slips for her previous partners.

Repeat cultures were taken two and three weeks later. These included rectal swabs, since 30% of treatment failures are detected from the rectum. Her results at follow-up were negative. Jenny was asked whether she had completed her medication, abstained from sex, informed her sexual partners and whether they were receiving treatment.

It is important to address a patient's emotional needs. Jenny was coming to terms with the infection and her partner was supportive and understanding. Reducing the risk of acquiring sexual infections in the future and the use of condoms was discussed, as were alternative methods of contraception.

References

Bignell, C. (1996) Antibiotic treatment of gonorrhoea – clinical evidence for choice. *Genito-urinary Medicine*; 72: 315–320.

Bingham, J.S. (1995a) Gonorrhoea now. *International Journal of STDs* and AIDS; 6: 3, 162–166.

Bingham, J.S. (1995b) Trends in female sexual behaviour and sexually transmitted disease in London, 1982–92. *Genito-urinary Medicine*; 71: 5, 286–290.

Communicable Disease Surveillance Centre/Public Health Laboratories. (1997) Sexually transmitted diseases among teenagers in England and Wales. *CDC Review*; 7: 12.

Daker-White, G., Barlow, D. (1997) Heterosexual gonorrhoea at St Thomas': patient characteristics and implications for targeted STD and HIV prevention strategies. *International Journal of STDs and AIDS*; 8: 2, 102–108.

Edwards, S., Carne, C. (1998) Oral sex and the transmission of non-viral STIs. *Sexually Transmitted Infections*; 74: 95–100.

Low, N., Daker-White, G., Barlow, D., Pozniak, A.L. (1997) Gonorrhoea in inner London: results of a cross-sectional study. *British Medical Journal*; 314: 1719–1723.

5. Genital herpes

Sue Chard

INTRODUCTION

Genital herpes is one of a number of viral infections that has increased in incidence within departments of genito-urinary medicine (GUM) in the last thirty years (Woolley, 1993). The sexual revolution of the 1960s produced a sharp rise in the number of cases of genital herpes, due partly to the introduction of the oral contraceptive pill (and therefore a reduction in the use of barrier forms of contraception), partly to increased social mobility (Hunt et al, 1993) and partly to a relaxation in attitudes towards sexual practices.

Today, great demand is put on the health care resources of GUM departments by patients with genital herpes needing to see a doctor, nurse or health adviser, sometimes on a number of occasions due to the recurring nature of the infection. Many patients are also seen in non-specialist centres such as at their local GP surgery, casualty department, or family planning clinics. In these centres it is important that the attending medical personnel are aware of current diagnostic techniques, new forms of treatment and the need to give appropriate counselling and advice to patients.

AETIOLOGY

In the 19th century some venereologists did not believe that genital herpes was sexually transmitted, or that women were often affected by the infection (Oriel, 1994). It was not until 1940 that Sharlit published an unequivocal report of one adult infecting another through sexual transmission.

We now know that genital herpes is caused by the herpes simplex virus (HSV), a member of the herpes virus family. Other 'relations' include *Varicella zoster* (also known as shingles or chicken pox), cytomegalovirus (CMV) and the Epstein-Barr virus.

There are two types of herpes simplex virus. Both types can cause genital infection, although HSV-1 is the usual cause of orolabial (facial) herpes, and HSV-2 is the cause of the majority of cases of genital herpes (Cunningham et al, 1997). The diagnosing of the HSV type is useful when discussing the likely prognosis of the infection with the patient. Patients infected with HSV-2 will usually have slightly more recurrences in the year following diagnosis of first-episode herpes than those infected with HSV-1 (Benedetti et al, 1994). To illustrate this, 95–98% of recurrent infection in GUM departments in Europe and Canada were shown to be HSV-2 (IHMF, 1997).

A typical evolving pathology of the infection is:

▶ cutaneous HSV exposure;

▶ acute infection (symptomatic or asymptomatic);

▶ recovery from acute infection;

▶ establishment of latent infection in the dorsal root ganglia, innervating the mucosal areas involved in acute infection;

▶ reactivation;

▶ release of virus from latently infected dorsal root ganglia;

▶ infection of epithelial cells, mucosal ulcerations;

▶ recurrent HSV – clinical or asymptomatic.

(adapted from Corey, 1994)

Latency is the time when the infection has gone into remission and viruses hide in nerves without replicating, i.e. the infection is not clinically apparent and the patient is asymptomatic. In a process that is not yet fully understood, the virus becomes reactivated and moves to the nerve endings and then into the epidermis or the oral or cervical/vulval mucosa, where it starts replicating and may cause a visible recurrence of the infection.

EPIDEMIOLOGY

HSV is a common genital infection. The number of first-episode HSVs reported by GUM clinics rose from 9593 (4519 men, 5074 women) in 1990 to 14,990 (5641 men, 9349 women) in 1996 (Simms et al, 1998). Studies have shown that around two-thirds of those with type-specific antibodies to HSV-2 have no apparent clinical symptoms (Cunningham et al, 1997). However, with education a significant number of these patients can be taught to recognise signs and symptoms of genital herpes.

Accurate figures are impossible to determine as patients are likely to attend their GP, A & E departments, or family planning clinics when complaining of genito-urinary symptoms, where there is not always the availability of the appropriate culture medium for diagnosis. Some people do not present at any medical facility. Also, only the results of first-episode genital herpes from GUM departments are included in the Communicable Disease Surveillance Centre's figures.

TRANSMISSION

The herpes virus is transmitted through direct skin-to-skin contact, usually between mucosal surfaces during genital-to-genital or genital-to-mouth contact. Transmission can occur when there are signs and symptoms of herpes. The ulcers that are typically present as a result of HSV infection contain viral infected fluid which, during oral, anal or vaginal intercourse can spread on to another person's skin. In more recent years, however, studies have shown that transmission can occur during sexual activity when there are no signs or symptoms of herpes being present (Cunningham et al, 1997). This is due to 'asymptomatic viral shedding' which, although not yet fully understood, has been suggested as the cause of the most frequent mode of transmission of herpes between sexual partners (Mertz et al, 1992). In the past, patients were advised that they were only at risk of passing the virus on during an outbreak of herpes and immediately before and after the outbreak. Now, the advice given to patients must sensitively and carefully reflect this new information.

SIGNS AND SYMPTOMS

First-episode HSV

After an incubation period of between two and fourteen days, first-episode HSV (also referred to as primary HSV) often presents as a severe illness with multiple genital ulcers. The symptoms cause varying degrees of pain, depending on the location and extent of the lesions, with women tending to experience the symptoms more severely. Most patients will present with dysuria, pruritis, enlarged and tender inguinal adenopathy and vaginal/urethral and, sometimes, anal discharge. There may be myalgia, arthralgia and a feeling of general malaise. The sites involved are the anogenital, cervical and urethral areas, with the vesicles on external genitalia (and occasionally the buttock and thigh) covering a large area of skin, with new sores appearing during the course of the infection. These vesicles often progress to form blisters that break, creating ulcers from which the herpes virus can be detected. These will then crust over on keratinised skin up to three weeks after the first vesicles have appeared.

In gay men who practise anal intercourse, primary herpes may cause anorectal pain, proctitis and tenesmus. In women the vulva may be oedematous and extremely sensitive, making insertion of a speculum impossible.

Passing urine over sores in the urethra and/or vulval area in women often causes pain. Men may also get dysuria if there are ulcers in the urethra. Understandably this causes some patients to avoid urinating, leading to retention. Very occasionally, urinary retention is due to the virus affecting the sacral autonomic plexus. However, with greater awareness of genital herpes by health care professionals and prompt commencement of antivirals, suprapubic catheterisation for this complication is now rarely seen. Neurological complications affect about 10% of patients with headaches, photophobia and viral meningitis (Adler et al, 1990). Due to the location of the sores, a secondary infection with either a fungus, or occasionally a bacterium, will occur.

Non-primary first-episode genital herpes occurs with milder symptoms than for primary HSV as the patient has serological evidence of a prior herpes infection (either HSV-1 or HSV-2).

Recurrent HSV episodes

In recurrent HSV episodes patients experience symptoms that are much less severe and shorter in duration, with fewer lesions that heal, on average, more quickly than those in the primary HSV outbreak (Adiman, 1994). There tends to be variability between each episode for an individual patient as well as between patients. Factors that appear to trigger the outbreak may be stress, friction, menstruation and conditions that compromise the immune system. More work needs to be done in this area to further our understanding. However, prodromal symptoms, or warning signs, are experienced by 50% of patients (Wilson, 1995) up to 48 hours before an HSV outbreak. The symptoms may be itching or tingling in the region where an outbreak may occur, sometimes accompanied by shooting pain down the leg, with or without hyperaesthesia of an area of the leg or buttock.

Atypical manifestations of herpes account for a large number of patients being under-diagnosed and misdiagnosed (Koutsky, 1992). The symptoms may include erythema and excoriations in women, and linear fissures and red spots on the glans of the penis in men.

Examination, diagnosis and tests

In first-episode genital herpes, the clinical diagnosis must be confirmed by a viral culture. A cotton wool swab should be rubbed over the lesions and, if any blisters are present, one should be broken open and swabbed (with goggles worn by the nurse or doctor). The swabbing will undoubtedly cause pain, but will hopefully pick up any viral fluid, which should be placed in a suitable HSV medium and kept at 4°C until transferred to the laboratory.

Direct immunofluorescence and enzyme-linked immunosorbent assays are sometimes used in the detection of HSV, with nucleic acid detection having the highest sensitivity, but its availability on the NHS is limited.

Unless it is too painful, a speculum examination should be performed on female patients and an HSV culture taken from the cervix. Male and female patients must have the standard sexually transmitted infection (STI) tests, including those for syphilis. Differential and concomitant diagnosis must always be considered.

When a patient presents with recurrent herpes, there is usually no systemic involvement. The pain is milder and more localised than with the primary outbreak. In female patients, blisters on the genitalia are common, but vulval soreness, itching, or something described as a "cut" can be present (Brocklehurst et al, 1993). Men often present with signs of recurrent non-specific urethritis, when in fact it is a urethral herpes infection that is causing the symptoms (Brocklehurst et al, 1993).

Psychosocial factors

Patient reactions to being told of a diagnosis of genital herpes vary. Some accept it as being a minor inconvenience, while for others, the chronic nature of the infection or the unpredictability of a recurrence means that a diagnosis may have a profound psychological effect (Dalkvist et al, 1995).

When first diagnosed with genital herpes, patients often show signs of emotional distress, depression (Bierman, 1983) and sometimes anger (Luby and Klinge, 1981). Many patients ask about possible treatments and a cure. Although there is antiviral therapy and a range of complementary choices for patients, there is no actual cure.

Patients have to cope with lesions on the most intimate part of the body, and often have fears about future outbreaks with the possibility of transmission of the virus to a present or future sexual partner. Some patients recall the scare-mongering in the 1980s that was reinforced by such phrases as "the sexual scourge" and the "curse of the promiscuous". As time goes on fewer will remember this, but while some do, perhaps it is not surprising that the infection is often associated with a great deal of stigma and embarrassment (Marchant and Roe, 1997). Research has shown a drop in sexual activity in at least 50% of patients with genital herpes (Bierman, 1983).

TREATMENT

First-episode HSV

Genital herpes is treated with an oral antiviral agent. Acyclovir, a nucleoside analogue, has been available as the only choice for over a decade. Recently, two new antiviral therapies, famciclovir and valaciclovir, have been introduced. Acyclovir acts on the herpes-infected cells by inhibiting the virus from making DNA and therefore preventing its viral replication. Although the two new antiviral drugs act in a similar way to acyclovir, they have better bioavailability. This means that, rather than taking the acyclovir five times a day, famciclovir can be taken three times a day and valaciclovir twice a day. This will hopefully ensure better patient compliance and hence improved treatment.

If a working diagnosis of first-episode HSV has been made, antiviral therapy should be started as soon as possible, as the drugs are most effective when used early on in an outbreak. This will reduce the severity of the symptoms (Russell, 1993).

The patient will usually be advised to take a mild analgesic for the flu-like symptoms and to rest for two to three days. The sores should be kept as clean as possible and can be bathed three to four times a day in a saline solution. If the patient is experiencing difficulties passing urine, he or she may find it easier to try to pass water in a warm bath. A topical anaesthetic may be prescribed to ease the pain.

Once told of the suspected diagnosis, the patient will require information on the virus, its transmission and prognosis. It is vital that time is spent with the patient at this point to explain and answer any questions he or she may ask. Patients may not remember all that is discussed on the first visit, so it can be helpful to provide written information to take away.

It may be appropriate to encourage the partner of the patient to attend the clinic for a physical examination and/or a discussion about the herpes virus and, although it may seem obvious, it is advisable to deter the patient from sexual intercourse until everything has healed.

As many patients are upset on hearing of the suspected diagnosis of genital herpes, the same health professional should see the patient on his or her follow-up if possible. This may be three to seven days later to give the patient results of any tests performed at the first visit and to ensure that no complications have arisen. This visit will allow the patient to ask further questions or have something confirmed, such as information on prodromes and how to recognise them.

If a speculum examination was not performed on female patients at the first visit, due to painful sores, it should be performed at the follow-up visit, and all the routine specimens taken for other STIs.

Recurrent episodes

If a patient presents with a (suspected) recurrence of genital herpes, depending on the circumstances, a detailed history may be required as to the frequency and severity of the recurrence(s) and what impact this is having on the patient's relationship and lifestyle. Where possible, the diagnosis should be confirmed by HSV culture, and tests taken for other STIs if appropriate.

Many patients prefer not to seek drug treatment for a recurrence of herpes, but for others it may be treated episodically as soon as they notice a prodrome or local symptoms. Some patients use complementary products such as *Echinacea purpurea*, a plant extract, tea tree oil and a range of other complementary therapies. Using cold tea bags on the sores, or gently drying them with a hair drier are methods sometimes used to encourage healing. The option of suppressive antiviral therapy should be made available to people who experience psychosocial, psychosexual or psychological disturbances associated with their frequent outbreaks of herpes. This may be for a short period of, for example, three months to cover a particularly important time, such as exams or a wedding, or it may be for longer. If the treatment is taken for longer, the patient would have three-monthly appointments to review the individual's situation, and six-monthly liver function tests to ensure that there were no long-term adverse effects. Suppressive therapy has a beneficial effect on quality of life (Carney et al, 1993).

Whichever form the treatment takes, the health professional must involve the patient, maintaining a non-judgmental approach and giving all current and relevant information to the patient. They will then, hopefully, come to a decision about the best treatment for that particular patient.

Allowing time to talk to the patient is not always easy, and in some clinics health advisers are employed specifically to allow patients further time to discuss issues around their diagnosis. Often, the health care professional will not be able to give a 'black and white' answer to patients' questions, but may suggest other reading material relating to genital herpes, or may suggest contacting the Herpes Association, whose telephone lines enable people to talk anonymously, at length if necessary, about worries they may have about herpes, thus providing psychological support and advice.

In the early 1980s it was often recommended that women with HSV infection have yearly cervical cytology performed. However, there is no evidence that HSV causes pre-cancerous changes in the cervix.

PREGNANCY

Patients often express concern about the risks associated with genital herpes in pregnancy. Neonatal herpes is seen in 1 in 60,000 to 70,000 live births in the UK (Stray-Pedersen et al, 1990) and results in infection of the neonate's eyes, mouth and skin. Worse cases present with encephalitis or disseminated infection which can lead to death of the neonate.

In the last few years, recommendations for the management of pregnant women with genital infection have been formulated by the Herpes Simplex Advisory Panel, a specialist interest group of the Medical Society for the Study of Venereal Diseases (MSSVD, 1998). Pregnant women should be asked about any history of genital herpes as part of their antenatal care. These women may be swabbed around the time of delivery to detect the virus. If the virus is detected immediately prior to delivery, or herpes ulceration is seen, the obstetrician will usually advise a Caesarean section. The most common time for the neonate to acquire the herpes virus is when it is in direct contact with the birth canal and virus-infected secretions (IHMF, 1997).

Where the mother has no herpes antibodies before pregnancy, and subsequently acquires first-episode genital herpes during pregnancy (especially in the third trimester) there is a higher relative risk of herpes transmission to the baby at delivery than if the mother had contracted herpes before pregnancy (Brown et al, 1991). First-episode genital herpes acquired during pregnancy also increases the risk of pre-term delivery (Stray-Pedersen et al, 1990).

Acyclovir is not licensed for use during pregnancy, but in some individual cases, in order to reduce the chance of viral shedding in women who experience frequent recurrences, obstetricians may wish to discuss the taking of acyclovir nearer to the time of delivery. Treatment with antivirals still presents a risk of neonatal mortality in babies with encephalitis or disseminated infection (Whitley et al, 1991).

CONCLUSION

New techniques in molecular biology have helped to rapidly improve our understanding of genital herpes. Research is now focusing on the less well-understood area of asymptomatic viral shedding and its relationship to transmission, and HSV-specific antibody testing. Vaccine studies are planned for the future.

While pharmaceutical companies continue to invest money in research and development of new herpes treatments, many patients now have a great interest in complementary therapies, some of which are currently being tested in clinical trials.

When discussing genital herpes, some patients will simply accept the diagnosis, while others will worry about future recurrences and other problems the infection may bring. Whatever the patients' response, our job as health care professionals is to provide them with correct up-to-date information and to give them time to express any anxieties and to ask questions.

Instead of focusing on worst case scenarios, which may encourage people to respond in a negative way, we must provide balanced information and carefully assess the individual holistically to achieve maximum physical and psychological health gain.

References

Adimora, A.A., Hamilton, H., Holmes, K.K. et al (1994) *Sexually Transmitted Diseases Companion Handbook.* New York: McGraw-Hill.

Adler, M.W. (1993) *ABC of Sexually Transmitted Diseases.* London: BMJ Publishing Group.

Benedetti, J., Corey, L., Ashley, R. (1994) Recurrence rates in genital herpes after symptomatic first-episode infection. *Annals of Internal Medicine*; 121: 847–854.

Bierman, S. M. (1983) Retrospective study of 375 patients with a history of genital herpes infections seen between 1973 and 1980. *Cutis*; 31: 5, 548–565.

Brocklehurst, P., Mindel, A. (1993) Recurrent genital infections. *British Journal of Sexual Medicine, Genital Herpes Compendium.*

Brown, Z.A., Benedetti, J., Ashley, R. et al (1991) Neonatal herpes simplex virus infection in relation to asymptomatic maternal infection at the time of labor. *New England Journal of Medicine*; 324: 18, 1247–1252.

Carney, O., Ross, E., Ikkos, G., Mindel, A. (1993) The effect of suppressive oral acyclovir on the psychological morbidity associated with recurrent genital herpes. *Genito-urinary Medicine*; 69: 6, 457–459.

Corey, L. (1994) The current trend in genital herpes. Progress in prevention. *Sexually Transmitted Disease*; 21: 2, 538–544.

Cunningham, A.H. (1997) *Clinician's Manual on Genital Herpes*. London: Science Press.

Dalkvist, J., Wahlin, T.B., Bartsch, E. et al (1995) Herpes simplex and mood: a prospective study. *Psychosocial Medicine*; 57: 2, 127–135.

Hunt, S., Kovachich, P., McKenna, S., et al (1993) Genital herpes and quality of life. *British Journal of Sexual Medicine, Genital Herpes Compendium*.

IHMF (International Herpes Management Forum) (1997) *The medical importance of genital herpes simplex virus infection*. Chapter 5, p.51. Recommendations from IHMF, 1997, XII Management Strategies Workshop 28th Feb – 1st March 1997, Sussex. U.K.

Koutsky, L.A., Stevens, C.E., Holmes, K.K. et al (1992) Underdiagnosis of genital herpes by current clinical and viral-isolation procedures. *New England Journal of Medicine*; 326: 23, 1533–1539.

Luby, E.D., Klinge, V. (1985) Genital herpes: a pervasive psychosocial disorder. *Archives of Dermatology*; 121: 4, 494–497.

Marchant, J., Roe, A. (1997) Genital herpes: recognizing and addressing patients' needs. *Herpes Journal*; 4: 36–41.

Mertz, G.J., Benedetti, J., Ashley, R. et al (1992) Risk factors for the sexual transmission of genital herpes. *Annals of Internal Medicine*; 116: 3, 197–202.

Oriel, J.D. (1994) *The Scars of Venus – A History of Venereology. Viruses and Chlamydia*. London: Springer-Verlag.

Russell, J. (1993) Diagnosis and management of recurrent genital herpes. *British Journal of Sexual Medicine, Genital Herpes Compendium*.

Sharlit, H. (1940) Herpes progenitalitis as a venereal contagion. *Archives of Dermatology*; 42: 933–936.

Simms, I. (1998) New cases seen at genito-urinary clinics in 1996. *Communicable Disease Report*. (Suppl) 8: S1–S11.

Stray-Pedersen, B., Bangstad, H.J., Bruu, A.L. et al (1990) Genital herpes in pregnancy. In: Guaschino, S. (ed.) *Infectious Diseases in Obstetrics and Gynaecology*. Bologna: Manduzzi.

Whitley, R.J., Arvin, A., Prober, C. et al (1991) A controlled trial comparing vidarabine with acyclovir in neonatal herpes simplex virus infection. *New England Journal of Medicine* ; 324: 7, 444–449.

Wilson, J.D. (1995) *Female Genital Infections: Infections of the Vulva.* London: Martin Dunitz.

Woolley, P. (1993) Introduction. *British Journal of Sexual Medicine, Genital Herpes Compendium.*

6. Genital warts

Tracy Wright

INTRODUCTION

Genital warts are caused by the human papilloma virus (HPV). They were
the most common sexually transmitted infection (STI) seen in genito-
urinary medicine (GUM) clinics in England and Wales in 1996 (Public
Health Laboratory, 1997) with 93,317 cases reported (Department of
Health, 1996). This number is believed to be underestimated as it excludes
patients who attend elsewhere or do not come forward for treatment.
There are now more than 80 types of HPV infection, with approximately
one-third affecting genital tissue. Genital infection can be clinical (warts),
subclinical (seen on cervical cytology or lesions only visible with
magnification) or latent (infection with apparently normal tissue) (Verdon,
1997). The transmission of genital HPV is nearly always by sexual contact
– autoinoculation from hands to genitals is unusual (Adler, 1995). The
exact pathogenesis of HPV remains uncertain. It is thought that the virus
gains entry into genital epithelium through tiny fissures and abrasions
caused by microtrauma sustained during sexual activity. The epithelial
cells then undergo a transformation and a wart is produced (Stedman,
1993). The infectivity of genital warts is approximately 60%, with an
incubation period of between two and eight months (average three
months) (Adler, 1995). For some people the virus may remain latent for
much longer than this.

SYMPTOMS AND DIAGNOSIS

Genital HPV can infect the squamous epithelia and mucous membranes of the cervix, vagina, vulva, penis, urethra, perineum and perianal region and may lead to the development of warts. These can appear as pink or fleshy lumps which are solitary or in clusters, and can be grouped into three generalised shapes: acuminata (pointed), papula (rounded), and macula (flat). In general warts are painless, but patients may complain of itching or tenderness and the warts may bleed after sexual intercourse. In women they are common at the posterior fourchette, vaginal introitus and adjacent labia and in men on the glans and shaft of the penis. Warts can affect any age group, but are most common in young sexually active individuals.

Diagnosis of visible warts is generally made in GUM clinics by clinical observation alone. Subclinical disease can be diagnosed with technical aids, e.g. a colposcope or histology. Latent disease will only be identified by detecting HPV DNA using a molecular biological technique in the laboratory, such as polymerase chain reaction (PCR). Prior to any genital examination, consent from the patient must be obtained and the procedure fully explained to him or her. Their privacy and dignity should be respected throughout. The genitalia should be examined in good clear light. In women a speculum examination may reveal warts on the cervix and vagina. Anal warts (that are not always associated with anal sex) can be seen using a proctoscope. Common anatomical variants of external genitalia and differential diagnoses that can be mistaken for warts need to be excluded. Approximately 25% of patients with genital warts will have a concurrent STI (Lacey, 1993), so it is therefore advisable to offer patients the full range of tests to screen for co-infections at initial diagnosis.

RISK FACTORS

Sexual activity, impaired cellular immunity and certain genetic host factors have been identified as important risk factors for HPV infection and HPV-associated neoplasias (Barrasso and Gross, 1997). Genital HPV can be grouped into low-, medium- and high-risk types in relation to their oncogenic potential (Barrasso and Gross, 1997). High-risk HPV types, particularly HPV 16, 18, 31 and 33, have been found in the majority of cervical cancers and cervical intraepithelial neoplasia (CIN) 3 lesions (Etherington, 1996). HPV types 6 and 11 (which are found in up to 95% of genital warts), are seen in low-grade CIN but rarely in cervical cancers (Verdon, 1997). Smoking is a co-factor for abnormal cervical cytology and the rate of progression of symptomatic HPV disease is increased in smokers (Feldman et al, 1997).

TREATMENT

There is no antiviral treatment available for HPV, therefore medical treatment is aimed at destroying the cosmetic disturbance the warts produce rather than killing the virus (McKeena, 1996). This is also important to help the patient's immune system fight the virus and to prevent further transmission. The outcome of wart treatment can be unsatisfactory, with high recurrence rates and prolonged therapeutic courses (Birley, 1994). This can be very frustrating for patients, causing them great anxiety. It is therefore essential that there is regular evaluation of treatment progress and that patients are kept informed and offered alternative treatment options as necessary. In the minority of cases warts may spontaneously disappear, but usually, if left untreated, they can grow in size and spread to other sites in the genital area (Hammond, 1995).

In some clinics, after their first visit and diagnosis, patients are able to have their treatment performed by a nurse. In the author's workplace, nurse-led wart treatment sessions are held where staff work within agreed departmental clinical guidelines. This has been found to allow a greater continuity of patient care and enhanced job satisfaction. Research has shown, from an audit of nurse-led wart clinics, that patient compliance improved due to flexible session times and shorter visits, and patients' waiting times were reduced (Frayne and Tobin, 1995).

Although there may be variations in clinical practice between clinics in the UK, the general principles of treatment are usually the same. Common treatments are podophyllin, podophyllotoxin and cryotherapy.

Podophyllin

Podophyllin is an established first line treatment for genital warts (White et al, 1997). It is a cytotoxic 10–25% topical solution in alcohol or benzoic solution. Treatment is clinic based and can be applied up to three times a week. The action of podophyllin results in acute destruction of the wart(s) over a few days, followed by healing. Careful application is required to avoid the development of chemical burns in the surrounding skin. The patient is instructed to wash the paint off in four to six hours to reduce skin soreness and irritation. Podophyllin cannot be used on cervical warts or broken skin. It is contraindicated in pregnancy due to its potential toxic and teratogenic effects, therefore any risk of pregnancy needs to be established.

Podophyllotoxin

Podophyllotoxin is the active ingredient of podophyllin. It is available in a stable chemical preparation in cream or solution for the home treatment of genital warts. Patients are assessed by a doctor for their suitability for this treatment and require careful instructions on usage to prevent over treatment and side effects occurring. It is useful for patients who have easily visible external warts, empowering them to take control of their own treatment. It also avoids repeated absences from work or disruption to the patient's lifestyle to attend clinic appointments. Although expensive, podophyllotoxin has been shown to be more cost effective than clinic-applied podophyllin, is superior in efficacy and has the potential to reduce the number of clinic visits (Kinghorn et al, 1993).

Cryotherapy

Cryotherapy is used to destroy warts by freezing them with liquid nitrogen, causing epidermal and dermal cellular necrosis (Lacey and Fairley, 1995). Liquid nitrogen can be applied with a cotton bud, spray gun or cryoprobe. Treatment can be painful for the patient and local anaesthetic cream may be prescribed to reduce this. Patients may complain of a 'burning' or 'frostbite' sensation during the freezing process. Care should be taking when freezing as localised oedema and inflammation occurs which, in some cases, can lead to severe ulceration. Patients should be given clear advice on skin care and pain control. Cryotherapy is useful for meatal, large or single warts.

Trichloracetic acid

Trichloracetic acid (TCA) is a caustic chemical solution applied directly to the wart(s) using a fine cotton bud, causing necrosis of superficial skin layers. Careful application is necessary to try and control the depth of tissue destruction in order to minimise ulceration and scarring. Patients usually experience burning at the site of application. TCA is useful for small, discrete or hyperkeratotic warts. No systemic toxicity occurs and the compound is not absorbed.

Electrocautery/hyfrecation

Electrocautery/hyfrecation is the use of a high frequency electric current from a wire electrode to destroy the wart(s). The procedure is performed by trained medical staff and requires a local anaesthetic. It is useful for large and solitary warts.

Less widely used treatments

Warts can be removed surgically under local or general anaesthetic using a sharp curette, scissors or a scalpel. Cervical warts can be treated with a carbon dioxide laser in gynaecology or colposcopy clinics. Fluoracil 5% gel can be used on external genitalia, but has common side effects of soreness, inflammation and severe chemical dermatitis with painful erosions. A recent development in HPV treatment is an immune response modifier called imiquimod (available as Aldara 5% cream). It is suitable for the home treatment of external and perianal warts and has been shown to be safe and effective with low recurrence rates. Interferons contain antiviral properties and can be administered topically or systemically. Systemic therapy can cause adverse reactions similar to non-specific viral symptoms. This is an expensive treatment and is not normally recommended for routine clinical practice as its efficacy is difficult to establish. At the present time there is no available therapeutic vaccine for HPV; research remains in the developmental stage.

PREGNANCY AND HPV

During pregnancy warts can increase dramatically in size, possibly due to depressed cellular immunity, and can regress quickly after delivery (Fong, 1994). Treatment during pregnancy is usually cryotherapy or TCA.

PATIENT INFORMATION AND CARE

A tactful and sensitive approach is essential when informing patients of their diagnosis. Unfortunately, the social stigma that still surrounds STIs often results in a range of negative feelings experienced by patients (Sheppard et al, 1995). Initial reactions can include feelings of shame, depression, isolation, anger and guilt (Clarke et al, 1996). In GUM clinics nurses or health advisers are available to provide psychological support and to discuss issues surrounding HPV. These include wart treatments, incubation period, HPV transmission, safer sex and partner notification. This information can be supported by a health education leaflet that the patients can take home with them to reiterate what has been said. Patients require information in relation to safer sex in order to reduce the risk of transmission of or reinfection with HPV. The effectiveness of using condoms to prevent transmission of HPV remains uncertain. It is thought that they may give some protection depending on the site of the warts. In one recent study it was found that clinics in the UK vary in the information they give about HPV and condom use, but the most common duration of time for condom use was for three months after the disappearance of the warts (Mclean and Hillman, 1997). Patients need to be advised about the importance of treatment compliance, potential side effects and the possibility of wart recurrence. Recurrence can be associated with a poor general immune system which may be caused by smoking, drugs, stress, immunosuppression and being HIV positive (Hammond, 1995). Women should be advised about the association between HPV and abnormal cervical cytology and also about the increased risk with co-factors such as smoking. At the present time there is a debate as to how often women with warts should have cervical smear tests performed, but women should be informed that they may have to have more frequent smears in accordance with the cytology department's policy. HPV typing can identify high-risk HPV in relation to cervical cancer, but this is currently not available on the NHS. The psychological effects that warts can have on patients should never be underestimated and can include impaired body image, and damaged self-esteem and self-confidence (Dudley, 1995). Research has shown that warts can negatively affect a patient's sexual activity and enjoyment (Clarke et al, 1996). It is therefore essential to offer patients support and health education at the time of diagnosis to try and reduce the occurrence of relationship problems and long-term psychological effects.

Reference

Adler, M.W. (1995) *ABC of Sexually Transmitted Diseases.* London: BMJ Publishing Group.

Barrasso, R., Gross, G. (1997) *Human Papilloma Virus Infection. A Clinical Atlas.* Berlin: Ullsten/ Mosby.

Birley, A. (1994) Podophyllotoxin, a better treatment for genital warts? *The Journal of Sexual Health.* April/May p42–45.

Clarke, P., Ebel, C., Catolti, D. et al (1996) The psychological impact of HPV infection. Implications for healthcare providers. *International Journal of STDs and Aids;* 7: 3, 197–200.

Department Of Health (1996) *STDs in England 1995. New cases seen at NHS GUM clinics.* London: DoH.

Dudley, W. (1995) The psychological impact of warts on patients' lives. *Professional Nurse;* 11: 2; 99–100.

Etherington, I., Shafi, M. (1996) Human papilloma viruses and cervical screening. *Genito-urinary Medicine;* 72: 3, 153–154.

Feldman, J., Chirgwin, K., Dehovitz., J. et al (1997) The association of smoking and the risk of *Condylomata acuminata* in women. *Obstetrics And Gynaecology;* 89: 3, 346–350.

Fong, R. (1994) Anogenital warts and their implications. *Maternal and Child Health;* August: 243–247.

Frayne, J., Tobin, J. (1995) An audit of nurse treatment sessions for female patients with genital warts. *International Journal of STDs and AIDS;* 6: 5, 363.

Hammond, J., Worlidge, P., Barton, S. (1995) Genital warts. *Practice Nursing;* 6: 2, 12–17.

Kinghorn, G.R., McMillan, A., Mulcahy, F. et al (1993) An open comparative study of the efficacy of 0.5% podophyllotoxin lotion and 25% Podophyllotoxin solution in the treatment of *Condylomata acuminata* in males and females. *International Journal of STDs and AIDS;* 414: 194 –199

Lacey, C. (1993) Genital warts and *Molluscum contagiosum. Medicine International;* 131–136.

Lacey, C., Fairley, I. (1995) Medical therapy of genital HPV-related disease. *International Journal of STDs and Aids;* 6: 6; 399–407.

McKeena, G. (1996) STDs: what's new? *Primary Healthcare New Zealand*; May p81–84.

Mclean, H., Hillman, R. (1997) Anogenital warts and condom use – a survey of information giving. *Genito-urinary Medicine*. 73; 203–206.

Public Health Laboratory (1997) *STDs Communicable Disease Report*; 7: 35; 310–311. London: PHLS

Sheppard, S., White, M., Walzman , M. (1995) Genital warts – just a nuisance? *Genito-urinary Medicine*; 71: 3, 194–201.

Stedman, Y. (1993) The management of genital warts. *British Journal of Sexual Medicine*; September/October, 20–24.

Verdon, M. (1997) Issues in the management of human papilloma virus genital disease. *American Family Physician*; 55: 5, 1813–1822.

White, D.J., Billingham, C., Chapman et al (1997) Podophyllin 0.5% or 2% v podophyllotoxin 0.5% for the self-treatment of penile warts. *Genito-urinary Medicine*; 73: 184–187.

7. Chlamydia

Annabel Davis

INTRODUCTION

Chlamydia is the most common curable sexually transmitted infection (STI) in the developed world (Taylor-Robinson, 1996). After the common cold, it is probably one of the most common human infections (Health Education Authority, 1992). Chlamydia is caused by the bacteria *Chlamydia trachomatis*, micro-organisms that live as parasites within a cell. It infects the genitals, and sometimes the eyes and throat.

Untreated chlamydial infections can have serious health consequences for both men and women. Thirty per cent of inadequately treated women will develop pelvic inflammatory disease (PID) (Stamm et al, 1984). More than half of these cases of PID are attributable to chlamydia (Westrom, 1980). Of these, 20% may become infertile and 10% will have an ectopic pregnancy (Johnson et al, 1996). Chlamydia is also the primary cause of epididymitis in young men (Rooney and Robinson, 1997).

Treatment of chlamydia is simple and effective, yet many cases remain undetected since up to 70% of women and 50% of men with the infection are asymptomatic (Cates and Wasserheit, 1991). Consequently, chlamydia is a major public health problem.

There are no national guidelines for the screening of chlamydia in the UK. However, the Department of Health set up an expert advisory group in 1995 to address screening issues. Other countries, notably Canada in 1989 and the USA in 1993, have issued national or selective screening guidelines for chlamydia. Major developments in the diagnosis and treatment of chlamydia in recent years have intensified the debate over screening and provided an impetus to improve recommendations for practice.

EPIDEMIOLOGY

There were 39,000 new cases of chlamydia in England and Wales in 1995, which was a 7% increase over 1994 (Department of Health, 1996). However, it is important to treat these figures with caution as they are only collected from genito-urinary medicine (GUM) clinics. Chlamydia is also treated in family planning clinics (FPCs) and private clinics, and by gynaecologists and general practitioners. Moreover, many cases are undetected because many asymptomatic people in sexually active populations do not seek health care (Holmes et al, 1990), so these figures are likely to underestimate the incidence of the disease.

The prevalence of chlamydia has never been comprehensively measured in the general UK population. Nevertheless, variable selection criteria have shown that between 2% and 12% of the population have chlamydia. The highest prevalence is among those aged under 25, and women who request a termination of pregnancy (Oakeshott and Hay, 1995).

In women, chlamydia usually presents as a cervical infection. In heterosexual men it is principally an infection of the urethra. It is rare in homosexual men as the pharynx and rectum are not easily infected, so only 2% of chlamydia is due to homosexual contact (Radcliffe, 1996). Between 30% and 50% of neonates born to women with untreated chlamydia will become infected with eye disease, and between 10% and 20% will contract pneumonia (Adler, 1995)

Finally, chlamydia can enhance the transmission of the human immunodeficiency virus (HIV) because the cervix is aggravated. For this reason, prevention of chlamydia can assist in the prevention of sexually transmitted HIV (Wasserheit, 1992).

SIGNS AND SYMPTOMS

Both men and women with chlamydia will present with symptoms similar to those of other STIs. In addition, chlamydia often occurs with a concurrent STI, in particular *Neisseria gonorrhoeae*.

Men may present with any combination of the symptoms outlined below:

- dysuria or frequency;
- a discharge from the penis, which may be clear, thin and milky-white in colour;
- burning and itching around the urethra;
- testicular pain, tenderness and swelling;
- lower abdominal pain or tenderness;
- an unusual discharge from the anus.

The urethra is the primary site of infection for 75% of male patients. However, chlamydia may ascend to the prostate, epididymis and the testes. It is also the most common cause of non-specific urethritis (NSU) in men.

Women may present with any combination of the symptoms outlined below:

- dysuria or frequency;
- a change in or an unusual vaginal discharge;
- lower abdominal pain;
- dyspareunia (pain on sexual intercourse);
- dysmenorrhoea, or disturbance of menstruation (for example, bleeding between periods);
- an unusual discharge from the anus.

Healthy vaginal secretions are clear, slightly milky or yellowish-white in colour, and have a faint, slightly musky odour. These vary between women and throughout the monthly cycle. It is important that women are aware of this in order to determine whether there is a change in their vaginal discharge (Furedi, 1992).

Chlamydia can also affect the upper genito-urinary tract and women may present with the associated symptoms of salpingitis (inflammation of the fallopian tubes), ectopic pregnancy (a pregnancy which occurs in blocked or inflamed fallopian tubes), or pelvic inflammatory disease (PID – infection and inflammation of the uterus, ovaries and the fallopian tubes, characterised by lower abdominal pain).

Pelvic inflammatory disease is an infection that ascends from the vagina, so the chances of getting PID are increased during the insertion of an intrauterine contraceptive device (IUD) (Murty, 1996) or following termination of a pregnancy (Thomas, 1997). It is most common in sexually active young women. The symptoms are:

- dyspareunia;

- dysmenorrhoea;

- fever and malaise;

- vaginal discharge – purulent cervical discharge;

- pain and tenderness on digital manipulation of the cervix.

The major implication of PID is infertility. The chances of infertility increase with each episode of PID – 10% after the first episode and 75% after the third episode (Adler, 1995). Other implications are ectopic pregnancy and associated psychological consequences.

EXAMINATION

To ensure an accurate diagnosis, a systematic process of investigation must be followed. Initially, an accurate history must be taken. A high-risk profile for chlamydia would contain the following (Adler, 1995):

- a change of partner;

- multiple sexual contacts;

- recurrent symptoms;

- symptoms in a partner;

- general symptoms (abdominal pain, menstrual problems, rash, dyspareunia, and arthralgia).

The physical examination must be comprehensive in case of a concurrent STI. For men the examination should include the penis, and the nurse should take a urethral swab and a urine sample. It is ideal if the urine is held for four hours prior to the examination to prevent the washing away of any specimens. The scrotum, pubic hair, surrounding skin and the perianal area should also be examined.

For women the examination should include the passing of a speculum to accurately visualise the cervix, the posterior fornix and the vagina. The cervix will sometimes bleed easily, show a purulent discharge and feel tender on swabbing. A specimen for chlamydia will be taken with a cotton-wool swab from the endocervix, the mucous membrane covering the neck of the uterus. The examination should also include taking swabs to eliminate concurrent STIs and a bi-manual examination of the vulva, pubic hair, surrounding skin and perianal area.

TESTING

Various methods are available for the diagnosis of chlamydial infection. The tests that are available have improved considerably over the last twenty years. The enzyme immunoassay (EIA) is frequently used, but the reliability of the test depends on a good specimen, so accuracy depends in part on the proficiency of the health practitioner taking the specimen. This test offers an approximate accuracy of 70%.

DNA amplification techniques are now available using a ligase chain-reaction (LCR) assay. The advantages of this test are that it can be done on urine and it is about 95% accurate. Although this test is twice as expensive as the EIA it detects considerably more cases (Lee et al, 1995).

However, no single test will identify all cases. Recent evidence shows that tests collected at home by women are as effective as those collected by GPs (Ostergaard et al, 1996). There is, however, still a need to evaluate women's attitudes to these screening methods. Decisions on which tests to use should be based on accuracy, cost and ease of collection.

PREGNANCY AND THE NEONATE

Chlamydia is transmitted to the neonate during the birth process. This can occur in two ways. The first is direct entry into the baby's eye during birth, which can cause eye disease and will affect 30–50% of neonates born to mothers with chlamydia. The second method of transmission is by the inhalation of infected material during birth, causing pneumonia. This will affect 10–20% of neonates born to mothers with chlamydia (Adler, 1995).

Eye disease will usually develop one to three weeks after birth and generally resolves spontaneously. However, in some untreated cases it will cause conjunctival scarring and micropannus formation. Although this condition is rare in the developed world, it is one of the leading causes of preventable blindness in the developing world (Hess, 1993).

Pneumonia or nasopharyngitis caused by the inhalation of infected material will develop in the first three months after birth.

TREATMENT

Treating adults is quite simple. The first choice of antibiotic has always been the tetracyclines – oxytetracycline or doxycycline (Adler, 1995). Erythromycin is effective for pregnant or lactating women, neonates and people who are intolerant of tetracyline. Both antibiotics are usually prescribed for a course of seven days.

Azithromycin has recently become available and can be taken as a single dose. It is as effective as doxycycline (Johnson et al, 1996), but costs twice as much. However, economic evaluations have shown azithromycin to be more cost-effective than doxycycline due mainly to greater compliance (Nuovo et al, 1995; Magid et al, 1996).

Women with PID should be prescribed oxytetracycline or doxycycline therapy for at least two weeks. In addition, they should be given a broad-spectrum antibiotic, such as metronidazole, which is also effective against *Neisseria gonorrhoeae* and other organisms. Bedrest or treatment as an inpatient may also be needed if the infection is severe.

Alternative remedies such as acupressure, Chinese herbs, herbal therapies and changes in diet can be effective, but it is important that antibiotics are taken. Alternative remedies are only used, after taking appropriate advice, to reduce symptoms and speed healing (Magid et al, 1996).

It is important that the patient tells their recent sexual partners to have a check-up, even if the partner is asymptomatic. Patients may find this subject difficult to broach with a partner – using a leaflet that provides information about chlamydia and its consequences can be one way of generating conversation with a partner. All sexual partners must be treated to prevent lasting damage to their reproductive system and to stop them from passing the infection on. Patients should be advised not to have sex until they are given the all-clear.

HEALTH EDUCATION AND HEALTH PROMOTION

It is important that people are made aware that chlamydia is transmitted during sex or birth but can be prevented through the use of barrier contraceptives, such as condoms. They should also be told that tests and treatment are simple and effective.

Access to services can be advertised through effective use of the media, sex education in schools and campaigns in the community.

Genito-urinary medicine clinics remain the best port of call, providing comprehensive tests, treatment and advice. Such clinics adopt an understanding and non-judgmental approach. Referral is not required and confidentiality is always respected, so anybody can attend for a check-up. Many GPs and FPCs will also perform the tests, but it has been argued that the role of GPs is suboptimal because inappropriate antibiotic treatment is sometimes given and partners are not always notified (Stokes, 1997). A recent family planning study showed a need for a more co-ordinated approach between health agencies in order to meet the needs of people using the services. There still seemed to be a reluctance on the part of GPs and FPCs to refer patients to GUM services (Thomas, 1997).

CONCLUSION

Chlamydia is a common and curable infection, but there is a need for increased awareness and screening. Raising awareness by introducing guidelines should improve detection rates and reduce the harmful effects of the infection. To achieve this various health agencies, including GPs, FPCs, GUM clinics and health promotion units must collaborate to set a complementary and unified agenda.

Case study

Melissa attended a local GUM clinic. She was seen by a doctor and explained that for the past two weeks her partner had had a penile discharge and discomfort while passing urine. He had attended his GP surgery, where he was advised to attend a GUM clinic. He had been diagnosed with non-specific urethritis, tested for chlamydia – for which he was still awaiting his results – given antibiotics and advised to ask his partner to attend for treatment and a check-up. The doctor then asked Melissa about her sexual and medical history.

Melissa was asymptomatic. She was aware of no change in her vaginal discharge and did not experience pain on passing urine or during sexual intercourse. Melissa and her partner had been having a relationship for four months and had used condoms for the first three months before Melissa started taking the Pill. It had been six months since she had had sex with anyone else. Her former partner, with whom she had a mono-gamous relationship for three years, was her only other sexual partner.

Melissa was visibly upset. She felt angry and confused, she said, because her current partner had told her that he had never slept with anyone else and she did not know whether to trust him anymore.

The doctor explained that the majority of women with chlamydia do not experience symptoms, but men are more likely to do so. Therefore, Melissa could have had the infection for a long time and not about known it. The doctor suggested that she have a full screen to test for chlamydia and to exclude any other sexually transmitted or genital infection at the same time. This would include a vaginal examination, blood tests and a internal digital examination.

After the examination, Melissa saw a health adviser who clarified several points. She said chlamydia is common, and explained the methods of transmission and the implications of leaving it untreated. She also stressed the importance of both partners taking antibiotics. Finally, the health adviser discussed the value of regular check-ups and the benefits of using condoms as a barrier to STIs.

Melissa said she felt a lot better now that she understood more about chlamydia. She felt less confused and more confident about discussing the situation with her partner.

Melissa then saw the doctor to get the provisional results of her exam-ination and to receive treatment. She felt a slight tenderness with digital manipulation of the cervix during the internal examination and her cervix bled a little when a swab was taken. However, there were no other signs of an STI. Melissa was given a one-week course of doxycycline to prevent re-infection and advised to abstain from sexual intercourse until the antibiotics were completed and both partners had clear negative results.

A week later Melissa received a positive chlamydia test result. She had completed her course of antibiotics and abstained from sexual intercourse. One week after that she and her partner reattended the clinic for repeat tests. Both were given the all-clear.

References

Adler, M.W. (1995) *ABC of Sexually Transmitted Diseases*. London: BMJ Publishing Group.

Cates, W., Wasserheit, J.N. (1991) Genital chlamydial infections: epidemiology and reproductive sequelae. *American Journal of Obstetrics and Gynaecology*; 164: 6, 1771–1781.

Department of Health (1996) *Sexually transmitted diseases, England 1995: new cases seen at NHS genito-urinary medicine clinics*. London: DoH.

Furedi, A. (1992) *Sexual well-being: a guide to intimate care for women* (a health promotion leaflet). London: Femidom Chartex.

Health Education Authority (1992) *Chlamydia and NSU: what they are and what you can do about them* (A health promotion leaflet). London: HEA.

Hess, D.L. (1993) Chlamydia in the neonate. *Neonatal Network*; 12: 3, 9–12.

Holmes, K.K., Mardh, P., Sparling, P.F. et al (1990) *Sexually Transmitted Diseases*. London: McGraw-Hill.

Johnson, A.M., Grun, L., Haines, A. (1996) Controlling genital chlamydial infection. *British Medical Journal*; 313: 7066, 1160–1161.

Lee, H.H., Chernesky, M.A., Schachter, J. et al (1995) Diagnosis of *Chlamydia trachomatis* genito-urinary infection in women by ligase chain reaction assay of urine. *The Lancet*; 345: 8944, 213–216.

Magdid, D., Douglas, J.M.J., Schwartz, J.S. (1996) Doxycycline compared with azithromycin for treating women with genital *Chlamydia trachomatis* infection: an incremental cost-effectiveness analysis. *Annals of Internal Medicine*; 124: 4, 389–399.

Mason, D., Kerry, S., Oakeshott, P. (1996) Postal survey of management of chlamydia infection in English and Welsh general practices. *British Medical Journal*; 313: 1193–1194.

Murty, J. (1996) Chlamydia: to screen or not to screen? One way to answer the question. *The British Journal of Family Planning*; 22: 3, 157–158.

Nuovo, J.N., Melnikow, Paliescheskey, M., King, J., Mowers, R. (1995) Cost-effectiveness analysis of five different antibiotic regimens for the treatment of uncomplicated *Chlamydia trachomatis* cervicitis. *Journal of the American Board of Family Planning*; 8: 1, 7–16.

Oakeshott, P., Hay, P. (1995) General practice update: chlamydia infection in women. *British Journal of General Practice*; 45: 400, 615–620.

Ostergaard, L., Moller, J.K., Anderson, B., Olesen, F. (1996) Diagnosis of urogenital *Chlamydia trachomatis* infection in women based on mailed samples obtained at home: multipractice comparative study. *British Medical Journal*; 313: 7066, 1186–1189.

Radcliffe, K. (1996) Chlamydia: testing for the silent threat to fertility. *Practitioner*; 240: 1561, 260–263.

Rooney, G., Robinson, A. (1997) Look out for the hidden STD. *Practitioner*; 241: 1576, 372–382.

Stamm, W.E., Guinan, M.E., Johnson, C. (1984) Effect of treatment regimens for *Neisseria gonorrhoeae* on simultaneous infection with *Chlamydia trachomatis*. *New England Journal of Medicine*; 310: 9, 545–549.

Stokes, T. (1997) Screening for chlamydia in general practice: a literature review and summary of the evidence. *Journal of Public Health Medicine*; 19: 2, 222–232.

Taylor-Robinson, D. (1996) Test for infection with *Chlamydia trachomatis*. *International Journal of STDs and AIDS*; 7: 1, 19–26.

Thomas, M. (1997) Chlamydia testing within family planning services: an audit of compliance with policies. *The British Journal of Family Planning*; 23: 92–95.

Wasserheit, J.N. (1992) Epidemiological synergy: interrelationships between human immunodeficiency virus infection and other sexually transmitted diseases. *Sexually Transmitted Diseases*; 19: 2, 61–77.

Westrom, L. (1980) Incidence and prevalence and trends of acute pelvic inflammatory disease and its consequences in industrialised countries. *American Journal of Obstetrics and Gynaecology*; 138: 7 (2), 880–892.

8. Vaginal thrush

Pippa Greer

INTRODUCTION

Vaginal candidiasis (thrush) is a major source of discomfort and inconvenience. It accounts for most complaints of vulvovaginal itching and irritation (Hamill and Kaufman, 1990) and it is one of the most common disorders for which women may seek medical attention.

Candida albicans is one of more than 80 species of candida and is the most common cause of vaginal candidiasis, with seven out of ten women experiencing at least one episode in their lives. The soreness and itching around the vulva and in the vagina may not be life threatening, but it can cause untold misery, dysuria and dyspareunia for many women, especially those who suffer from repeated episodes (Dulfer, 1989).

EPIDEMIOLOGY

Vaginal thrush is invariably caused by *candida albicans*, a yeast that normally lives unobtrusively in the gut, mouth and genital tract. The yeast usually lives in ecological balance with the normal commensal flora. *Candida albicans* is a Gram-positive fungus. It is a unicellular organism and demonstrates a filamentous growth. The fungus reproduces sexually by producing spores, or asexually by budding.

Thrush can occur in both males and females and among all age groups, in those groups who may be sexually active and those who are celibate.

Candida thrives in a warm, moist and dark environment and will proliferate when its habitat becomes altered. The vagina is therefore an ideal host for such an infection.

Most women may carry candida without experiencing the symptoms of thrush. It may not cause symptoms due to the vagina's natural defence mechanism. For symptoms to develop, the candida must become activated and increased in number. Two of the factors that contribute to the vagina's defence mechanism are lactobacilli and pH.

Lactobacilli

Lactobacilli are Gram-positive bacteria that inhabit the vagina as part of its natural flora. They have the ability to convert glycogen into lactic acid, therefore inhibiting fungal growth.

pH

The normal pH of the vagina is 4.5, which is slightly acidic and will therefore also keep certain organisms at bay. The pH is crucial to the homeostasis of the vagina. Any changes in the vaginal pH or any excess unconverted glycogen will, therefore, automatically predispose to thrush.

PREDISPOSING FACTORS

An example of some of the factors that may cause a change in vaginal pH are: semen, menstrual blood, perfumed soaps, feminine hygiene products and douching.

In pregnancy and premenstrually, the sex steroid receptors act on the yeast to accelerate growth, i.e. the rise in hormone levels causes excess glycogen to be excreted – too much for the lactobacilli to convert into lactic acid. In pregnancy thrush does not cause a risk to the foetus and is not an indication for Caesarean section.

The older contraceptive pills containing higher doses of oestrogen were at one time associated with recurrent thrush, but the third generation pill is not considered a risk factor (Bowman, 1992).

Stress can trigger increased amounts of adrenaline, which in turn will affect our sex hormones, which may lead to changes in the menstrual cycle, therefore altering the pH balance of the vagina.

If the vulva and the vagina become excessively warm and moist as a result of wearing nylon tights, man-made fibres and tight fitting clothes, thrush again will proliferate.

Other predisposing factors include tampons (which are thought to change the normal vaginal ecology) and excess dairy products, sucrose, artificial sweeteners, wine and coffee, which all lead to an increase in urinary sugar, therefore providing nourishment for the yeast. Sugars also have the effect of lowering the body's natural immunity.

The yeast organism acts like any other infectious agent on the host. The virulence of the agent and the resistance of the host are important factors. The resistance of the host, in this case the vagina, is altered by the immune system of the body. So, individuals who are prescribed corticosteroids, are on immuno-supressant therapy or who may be HIV positive, will be predisposed to thrush.

Women who use a contraceptive intra-uterine device may also be predisposing themselves to candidal infection, as residual candida spores have been isolated on the threads of the device.

Finally, antibiotics, diabetes, trauma, reduced lubrication and anaemia are also considered to be predisposing factors.

SIGNS AND SYMPTOMS

These may vary greatly with each individual. Some women may present with a normal, healthy-looking vagina and vulval area, while others may present with obvious oedema and erythema. This is due to the overgrowth of the yeast, giving rise to an inflammatory response.

The most common and often the most distressing symptom is itching and soreness around the vulva and inside the vagina. Vaginal discharge may also be present, often described as 'cottage cheese-like' in appearance: thick and white, often seen in plaques adhering to the vaginal walls. Creamy discharge, and even an absence of discharge, have also been described.

Other symptoms may include dysuria (pain and difficulty in passing urine), possibly due to the urine coming into contact with the inflamed skin of the vulva; and dyspareunia (painful sex), caused by the inflammatory response or lack of lubrication.

It is imperative to acknowledge that the symptoms may not necessarily be indicative of candida, but may be signs of other common genital infections. It is essential that an accurate diagnosis is made, with the assistance of appropriate history taking, examination and tests.

In a male the signs and symptoms may present as a rash and itching, accompanied by some dysuria and possibly superficial ulcers. Once again it is essential that an accurate diagnosis is made.

TRANSMISSION

Human beings are the major source of candida infection in other human beings. The yeast, as previously discussed, has been isolated from the mouth, vagina, rectum and under the foreskin of an uncircumcised male. The incubation period from potential infection is two to five days. The organism may be transmitted via sexual intercourse, during foreplay by fingers and oral–genital contact. Men are most likely to acquire thrush during sex. In women it is generally linked with predisposing factors and alterations in the body's natural defence mechanism.

DIAGNOSIS

Diagnosis can differ greatly between different practitioners. Ideally diagnosis should take place in a genito-urinary medicine (GUM) clinic. Some GPs and family planning clinics may have suitable facilities.

History

Accurate history taking is essential. Factors that must be discussed and documented include signs and symptoms, for example, is there any abnormal discharge, pain when passing urine or having sex. The duration of the signs and symptoms and how often they occur should also be considered, for example, does it occur every month just before a menstrual period. There should also be discussion around predisposing factors, for example, family history of diabetes or recent antibiotic therapy.

CLINICAL DIAGNOSIS

On examination of the vulva and the vagina, loss of natural lubrication, and/or excessive white discharge may be noted, together with a change in the colour and texture of the labia. This may appear shiny, pink or red and inflamed.

In a GUM clinic, a full bacteriological examination will take place. Specimens will be collected from the lateral vaginal walls, endocervix, posterior fornix and the urethra in a female patient and from beneath the foreskin, sub-prepuce, and the urethra in a male patient.

A specimen of vaginal discharge from the lateral vaginal walls will be collected with the appropriate materials for microscopy. A specimen for culture will be sent to the laboratory; this will enable the bacteriologists to identify and isolate any pathogenic organisms.

A sample of discharge from the posterior fornix, an area just below the cervix, where secretions pool, should be taken for a wet preparation slide. Normal saline is used to prepare this wet mounted slide. On reading the slides under the microscope (microscopy) spores and/or hyphae will be seen if candida infection is present. Microscopy has been reported as only 50% accurate, therefore culture may also be used as it is considered to be far more precise. Sabouraud culture plates and Feinberg Whittington media are the most commonly used. Bacterial swabs sent for microscopy, culture and sensitivity may also grow candida and assist in the detection of the species of the organism present.

A full bacteriological screen will eliminate other pathogens, for example bacterial vaginosis, *Trichomonas vaginalis*, *Neiserria gonorrhoeae* and other common genital infections that may present with a similar history.

If no spores or hyphae are seen on initial microscopy, but the historical and clinical findings are indicative of candidiasis, then most clinicians will offer treatment.

TREATMENT

There are several treatments available, both traditional orthodox methods and complementary methods.

Traditional treatment options

The most widely used traditional form of treatment is with an antifungal agent, such as clotrimazole. A combination of vaginal pessaries and topical cream may be used, for example, clotrimazole 200mg pessaries inserted into the vagina at night for three consecutive nights in conjunction with a topical application of 20g of 1% clotrimazole cream to the external genitalia. Clotrimazole 500mg pessary as a one-off treatment is also used. This method of treatment can feel 'gritty' and can be slow to work, so it is essential that the patient be informed that there may not be an immediate response, and that symptoms may not resolve for two to three days. Clotrimazole 10g intravaginal cream is another form of anti-fungal treatment and is often preferred by clinicians if there is no vaginal discharge present.

No systemic toxic effects have been reported with any of the treatments mentioned above. Despite these treatments being readily available over the counter, they may not necessarily be appropriate unless an accurate diagnosis has been made.

Male patients may be treated with a topical application of clotrimazole cream, 20g of 1%, twice a day for three days.

Fluconazole (Diflucan) 200mg may be given as a stat dose orally. However, this treatment is not recommended if there is a risk of pregnancy.

Health education is of paramount importance. Discussion must take place about the effects of predisposing factors, for example perfumed soaps, or diet.

Treatment of relapsing infection

Many women will not have one isolated case of vaginal thrush, but will suffer from recurrent episodes. When a female patient reattends, then an accurate history and examination should take place as previously discussed. It is also an ideal opportunity to evaluate, where possible, if any changes in behaviour have been made in relation to predisposing factors, and if the patient understands why she may have a predisposition to thrush. At this point it may be appropriate to instigate further medical tests to provide evidence for concurrent or undiagnosed disease, for example, a sample of blood may be taken and tested for blood sugar levels and/or anaemia, as these two factors are known to predispose to thrush.

A prolonged course of treatment is sometimes advised when patients keep reattending, for example, clotrimazole 100mg pessary for 12 days. This method tends not to be very popular. Prophylactic treatment may also be offered in some cases and this takes the form of one 500mg pessary one day a week or one day a month for two to three months.

Finally, it is often useful to establish if the male partner has been treated concurrently. Even though candida is not considered to be a sexually transmitted infection, it is known that it may be transmitted between partners if one partner remains untreated.

Alternative treatment options

A number of alternative or complementary therapies have been thoroughly researched. Some examples are:

> The tea tree plant is known to produce one of the most medicinally active essential oils, which in recent years has gained increasing recognition from orthodox medical practitioners and complementary therapists. The tea tree plant is indigenous to Australia and is from the same family as the eucalyptus.

> Tea tree oil may be used in a variety of ways. Prophylactically eight to ten drops may be added to a bath. Alternatively a tampon may be soaked in a 1% solution of tea tree oil and purified water (20 drops to 100mls) before being inserted into the vagina (Lawless, 1994).

> Patients opting for this method of treatment must be advised that, although it is normal to experience a temporary warm sensation when tea tree oil is used in the vaginal area, treatment must be discontinued immediately if burning or irritation develops.

> There have been several studies evaluating the use of live natural yoghurt as a means of prophlyaxis (Hilton et al, 1992). The yoghurt must contain *Lactobacillus acidophilus*. It can either be ingested on a regular basis or, once again, used in conjunction with a tampon. The top section of the tampon may be filled with the live natural yoghurt and inserted into the vagina, the tampon can be removed and the yoghurt will stay in position.

> A study in 1990 demonstrated that if damp, freshly laundered underwear is microwaved for five minutes, the candida spores will be

killed. If the underwear is freshly laundered and dry the spores remain even after thirty minutes in a microwave (Phillips and Friedrich, 1990).

▷ Garlic is a powerful natural antibiotic. Whole cloves of garlic may be inserted into the vagina, but a more preferable method is to use odourless garlic supplements orally.

▷ The Chinese believe that illness comes from within. Therefore, they believe that our health is determined by our ability to maintain a balanced internal environment. Acupuncture is believed to achieve this.

▷ *Lactobacillus acidophilus*, *bulgarus* and *bifidus* taken three times a day, between meals, has been recommended as a prophylactic measure. The rationale for taking the supplements between meals is that the digestive juices will not interfere with absorption.

▷ Sugar, monosodium glutamate, smoked fish, sausages, vinegar, coffee, yeast and cheese are several of the foods that it is recommended to avoid in order to prevent predisposition to recurrent candidiasis.

It is important to remember that a systematic and logical approach is required in order to help patients remain symptom free, and that patients may require a sensitive, psychological approach to assist them in overcoming their discomfort and to prevent their own distress about the condition actually becoming a predisposing factor in itself.

Case study

The following scenario focuses on health education following a diagnosis of candida within an STI setting (GUM clinic). The patient-directed educational approach was used throughout.

Hannah, a 24-year-old woman, presented to the clinic for the third time in a six-month period, with a history of soreness and itching around her vulva and in her vagina. On each attendance she was diagnosed as having 'thrush'.

Hannah was in a regular relationship and used condoms as a means of contraception.

The meeting took place opportunistically in one of the clinical rooms. Hannah had several questions following her diagnosis: was her partner to blame? Why did the symptoms develop just before her period was due? What other treatments were available apart from pessaries?

The nurse reassured her that thrush was not considered to be a sexually transmitted infection. However, it was possible that, if her partner was not treated and they had unprotected sex, the thrush could pass backwards and forwards between them. However, this mode of transmission seemed unlikely as they never had unprotected sex and had not experienced any broken condoms.

Hannah had, for a time, marked in her personal diary when she was getting sore and itchy and noticed that it was several days before her period was due. The nurse explained that there are increased levels of hormones released at this time, and that the vagina's defence mechanism might be unable to cope with converting all the excess glycogen into lactic acid. Hannah had also requested information about alternative treatments, so she was told that she could try using live natural yoghurt on a tampon as a means of prophylaxis.

Hannah was given a contact name and telephone to call if she thought of anything else she wanted to ask once she left the department. She was also given a leaflet as a back up.

Hannah telephoned the clinic several months later to thank staff for their advice. She had not experienced any further episodes of thrush before her period and was very grateful for the advice that she had received.

It is worth mentioning at this point that such a quick resolution may not always occur, and that perseverance with the avoidance of predisposing factors and investigation into undiagnosed disease may be time consuming but is necessary.

References

Adler, M.W. (1995) *ABC of Sexually Transmitted Diseases.* London: BMJ Publishing Group.

Bowman, C.A. (1992) Recurrent vulvovaginal candidosis. *British Journal of Sexual Medicine;* 19: 5,133–36

Dulfer, S. (1989) Vaginal thrush. *Practice Nurse;* 2: 3, 105.

Hamill, H., Kaufman, R.H. (1990) Vaginal candidiasis: tailoring the treatment. *Physician Assistant*; 14: 7, 41–44.

Hilton, E., Isenberg, H.D., Alperstein, P., et al (1992) Ingestion of yoghurt containing *Lactobacillus acidophilus* as prophylaxis for candidal vaginitis. *Annals of Internal Medicine*; 116: 5, 353–357

Lawless, J. (1994) *Tea Tree Oil. A new guide to one of Nature's most remarkable gifts.* London: Thorsons.

Phillips, L.E., Friedrich, E. (1990) Microwaving underwear. *American Journal of Nursing*; 90: 9, 17.

9. Bacterial vaginosis

Lovelle Smith

INTRODUCTION

Bacterial vaginosis (BV) is a common vaginal infection that affects 12–20% of women of reproductive age (McDonald et al, 1997). There is an ongoing debate over whether transmission during sexual intercourse is a causal factor, and research indicates that it is also common in women who have sex with women (McCaffrey et al, 1997).

The infection is associated with pelvic inflammatory disease (PID) (Sweet, 1987) cervical intra-epithelial neoplasia (CIN), infertility and spontaneous preterm delivery and labour.

Women with BV have distinct changes in vaginal flora, with an associated elevated vaginal pH, growth of pathogenic flora and, in some cases, homogeneous, malodorous discharge (Eschenbach, 1993). The misconception that the unpleasant odour is due to poor hygiene can result in anxiety for women with BV intending to seek medical treatment.

HISTORY OF BACTERIAL VAGINOSIS

Lactobacilli were first discovered in 1894, by Doderlein, as the main organism in 'normal' vaginal flora. In the study, vaginal flora were considered to be homogeneous and consisting only of lactobacilli. Abnormal vaginal flora were heterogeneous, with an absence of lactobacilli. The term non-specific vaginitis was used to describe the infection.

In 1955 Gardner and Dukes isolated an organism that they believed caused non-specific vaginitis. The organism was called *Haemophilius vaginalis*, and the infection was renamed *Haemophilius vaginalis* vaginitis (Eschenbach, 1993). In 1963, the organism was renamed *Corynebacterium vaginalis* and in 1980 it was renamed again to *Gardnerella vaginalis*, in honour of Dr Gardner, and the infection became known as *Gardnerella vaginalis* vaginitis.

With the development of sophisticated laboratory techniques, it became apparent that *Gardnerella vaginalis* is present in more than 50% of asymptomatic women and that more than one type of bacteria is implicated in the infection (Eschenbach, 1993). During the 1980s it became evident that anaerobic bacteria were responsible for the fishy odour, and the infection became known as anaerobic vaginosis.

In 1984, the name bacterial vaginosis was coined, to reflect the many different types of bacteria involved and the lack of vaginal inflammation with the condition (Morse et al, 1996).

AETIOLOGY

It is now agreed that BV is a change in the vaginal environment from having 'normal' acid-producing lactobacilli flora, to mixed anaerobic flora. This can be characterised by an increase in vaginal discharge, a pH elevated above 4.5, the production of amines resulting in a fishy odour (Morse et al, 1996; Ison, 1997) and clue cells on microscopy.

Clue cells (Gardner and Dukes, 1955; Amsel et al 1983) are epithelial cells that are covered with mixed flora organisms. The mixed flora obscure visibility of the cell wall, resulting in a salt-and-pepper appearance during microscopic examination.

The fishy odour is caused by the production of volatile amines released by the bacteria (Morse et al, 1996) and not, as is sometimes believed, poor hygiene.

SIGNS AND SYMPTOMS

Women with BV may complain of an increased, milky, foul smelling discharge, but this is not always the case as some women are asymptomatic. In symptomatic women, 90% will complain of a vaginal discharge and over 70% will complain of an odour (Morse et al, 1996).

CAUSES

The exact cause of BV is unknown. However, some suggested causes are genetic factors, vaginal douching, the use of scented soaps and bath additives, residual semen after unprotected sexual intercourse and hormonal changes during the menstrual cycle (Keane et al, 1997a; Taylor-Robinson and Hay, 1997).

PREDISPOSING FACTORS

Some researchers argue that BV is a sexually transmitted infection and that it occurs frequently in women who are very young at first coitus and who have many sexual partners (Larsson et al, 1991). However, no study has documented that the treatment of male sexual partners reduces the incidence of BV .

The infection has been isolated in virgins (Bump and Buesching, 1988) and some studies conclude that unprotected sexual intercourse may help to resolve BV in some women (Hay et al, 1997).

A recent study by Keane et al (1997b) indicates an association between non-gonococcal urethritis (NGU) and BV. The study suggests that when the large numbers of the bacteria in BV are present, they may cause NGU in male partners. This suggests that BV is sexually transmissible, but not exclusively a sexually transmitted infection.

In spite of the contrasting views of researchers, women attending genito-urinary medicine (GUM) clinics are told that BV is not a sexually transmitted infection and their partners are not routinely screened and treated.

Black women are believed to be at increased risk of BV, and there is evidence that they have a higher incidence of the infection (Llahi-Camp et al, 1997). Some of the reasons suggested for this are that black women have a genetically elevated vaginal pH and that the practice of vaginal douching, which is more common among black women, may have a detrimental affect on 'normal' vaginal flora.

DIAGNOSIS

The standard diagnostic criteria used today for the detection of BV was developed by Amsel et al, in 1983. A diagnosis of BV can be established by identifying the presence of any three of the four following signs:

- a positive whiff test;

- an elevated vaginal pH (above 4.5);

- clue cells on microscopy;

- a thin, homogeneous vaginal discharge.

Women attending a GUM clinic will have a speculum examination, when a sample of vaginal secretions from the vaginal walls is taken. In symptomatic women, on speculum examination, a grey, milky discharge that clings to the vaginal walls can be seen and there is an absence of inflammation, which led to the term vaginosis rather than vaginitis (Morse et al, 1996). Sometimes the vaginal secretions can be smelt when withdrawing the speculum and, because normal secretions do not have an odour, this may indicate a positive result.

A more sensitive whiff test that can be carried out is performed by the addition of a few drops of 10% potassium hydroxide solution to the vaginal secretion sample, and is smelt immediately. The potassium hydroxide is an alkaline solution, which allows the release of volatile amines, resulting in the characteristic fishy odour. Recent health and safety issues concerning the whiff test have resulted in a study examining the use of a weaker strength potassium hydroxide. The results that were presented at a 1998 BV conference indicate that 1%, or even 0.1%, is equally sensitive and safer to use in a clinical environment.

The pH of the vaginal secretions is determined by using a strip of litmus paper, which is sometimes placed directly on to the vaginal wall or on to the withdrawn speculum. Care must be taken not to sample cervical secretions and the water used to lubricate and warm the speculum, as these have a pH of around seven.

Clue cells are epithelial cells covered with mixed anaerobic flora, to the extent that the cell wall is not clearly visible. A vaginal sample should be taken and placed on a drop of saline on a slide. The drop should be covered with a cover slip and microscopically examined for the presence or absence of clue cells. Women without BV have epithelial cells with clear borders and the presence of lactobacilli (Morse et al, 1996).

The Gram-stain method of diagnosis is also used, in conjunction with Amsel et al's (1983) diagnostic criteria. A vaginal sample is taken and placed on a slide. The slide is then heat-fixed, Gram-stained and microscopically assessed for the presence of clue cells and absence of lactobacilli.

TREATMENT

BV is known to spontaneously resolve in some women. However, the drug of choice is the antibiotic metronidazole, taken for five days, which has a 99% cure rate. Metronidazole is contraindicated during the first trimester of pregnancy, because of concerns of potential carcinogenicity. It can, however, be used in the second trimester.

More recently, some studies indicate that vaginal clindamycin cream is the best treatment for BV and claim cure rates of 90% after one week (Larsson, 1997). Vaginal clindamycin is the preferred treatment during the first trimester and early second trimester of pregnancy (Dennemark et al, 1997).

Some clinicians prescribe preparations that attempt to reintroduce the acid-producing lactobacilli to the vaginal environment. Treatments such as yoghurt, lactic acid gel, acetic acid gel and hormonal creams have been used, but in controlled studies their affects have been found to be nothing more than placebo (Morse et al, 1996).

Recent data presented at a 1998 BV conference state that tee tree oil gel can also be used vaginally to treat BV.

CONCLUSION

Bacterial vaginosis is an infection that affects a large number of women of reproductive age. The infection has been associated with serious gynaecological and obstetric complications, which advocates the screening and treatment of women of reproductive age prior to pelvic surgery, when presenting with vaginal symptoms and at antenatal visits.

Although the infection can spontaneously resolve and return, both increased nursing and client awareness, and clarity concerning the mechanisms of transmission are needed.

Case study

Affela was a 24-year-old woman who attended a genito-urinary clinic in London. She complained of an offensive vaginal discharge, which had started five days previously and had not improved. She said she did not feel sore or itchy but, because of the foul discharge, she had been adding a scented disinfectant to her bath. Initially, she thought she had vaginal candidiasis and had used clotrimazole pessaries, but her symptoms had not disappeared.

The symptoms appeared to worsen after sexual intercourse and she attended the clinic for diagnosis and treatment after her partner complained about the fishy smell.

Her last period had been approximately two weeks prior to the visit and she used the Pill as a contraceptive.

During the speculum examination, Affela was very nervous and continually apologised for the offensive smell. Swabs for microscopy and culture were taken for chlamydia, gonorrhoea, trichomonas, candida and bacterial vaginosis.

There was a positive whiff test and clinical findings established the presence of clue cells on microscopic assessment and a vaginal pH of six.

A diagnosis of bacterial vaginosis was made and Affela was prescribed 500mg of metronidazole tablets twice daily for five days.

A nurse gave Affela her medication and a leaflet about the infection. Methods of avoiding further reinfection were discussed, and she was advised to return to the clinic if her symptoms persisted or worsened.

References

Amsel, R., Totten P.A., Speigel, C.A. et al (1983) Non-specific vaginitis. Diagnostic criteria and microbial and epidemiologic associations. *The American Journal of Medicine;* 74:15–21.

Bump, R.C., Buesching, W.J. (1988) Bacterial vaginosis in virginal and sexually active adolescent females: evidence against exclusive sexual transmission. *American Journal of Obstetrics and Gynaecology;* 158: 4, 935–939.

Dennemark, N., Meyer-Wilmes, M., Schluter, R. (1997) Screening and treatment of bacterial vaginosis in the early second trimester of pregnancy: a sufficient measure for prevention of preterm deliveries? *International Journal of STDs and AIDS;* 8: 1, 38–40.

Doderlein, A. (1894) Die scheidensekretuntersuchugen. *Zentralts Gynakol;* 18: 10–14.

Eschenbach, D.A. (1993) History and review of bacterial vaginosis. *The American Journal of Obstetrics and Gynaecology;* 169: 2, 441–445.

Gardner, H.L., Dukes, C.D. (1955) Haemophilius vaginalis vaginitis. A newly defined specific infection previously classified 'non-specific' vaginitis. *The American Journal of Obstetrics and Gynaecology;* 69: 962–976.

Hay, P.E., Ugwumadu, A., Chowns, J. (1997) Sex, thrush and bacterial vaginosis. *International Journal of STDs and AIDS;* 8: 1, 603–608.

Ison, C.A. (1997) Microbiology and Epidemiology: Introduction. *The International Journal of STDs and AIDS;* 8: 1, 2–3.

Keane, F.E., Ison, C.A., Taylor-Robinson, D. (1997a) A longitudinal study of vaginal flora over a menstrual cycle. *International Journal of STDs and AIDS* 8: 1, 489–494.

Keane, F.E., Thomas, B., Renton, A. et al (1997b) Investigation into a possible causal role of bacterial vaginosis in non-gonococcal urethritis. *Genito-urinary Medicine;* 73: 5, 373–377.

Larsson, P.G., Platz-Christensen, J.J., Sundstrom, E. (1991) Is bacterial vaginosis a sexually transmitted disease? *International Journal of STDs and AIDS;* 2: 5, 362–364.

Larsson, P.G. (1997) Treatments for bacterial vaginosis: an update on the expected cure rate. *International Journal of STDs and AIDS;* 8: 1, 35–36.

Llahi-Camp, J.M., Ison, C.A., Regan, L. et al (1997) The association between bacterial vaginosis and infertility. *International Journal of STDs and AIDS*; 8: 1, 23–24.

McCaffrey, M., Varney, P.A., Evans, B. et al (1997) A study of bacterial vaginosis in lesbians. *International Journal of STDs and AIDS* 8: 1, 11.

McDonald, H.M., O'Loughlin, J.A., Vigeneswaran et al (1997) Metronidazole treatment of bacterial vaginosis flora and its effect on preterm birth. *International Journal of STDs and AIDS*; 8: 1, 37–38.

Morse, S.A., Moreland, A.A., Holmes, K.K. et al (1996) *CD-Atlas of Sexually Transmitted Diseases and AIDS*. London: Mosby International.

Sweet, R.L. (1987) Pelvic inflammatory disease and infertility in women. *Infectious Disease Clinicians North America*; 1: 99–125.
Taylor-Robinson, D., Hay, P.E. (1997) The pathogenesis of the clinical signs of bacterial vaginosis and possible reasons for its occurrence. *International Journal of STDs and AIDS*; 8: suppl. 1, 13–16.

10. Trichomoniasis

Annabel Davis

INTRODUCTION

Infection due to *Trichomonas vaginalis* (TV) is the most common non-viral sexually transmitted infection (STI) in the world (Petrin et al, 1998), yet this non-lethal pathogen has received relatively little attention, reflected by the lack of widely published information. However, this may change since recent research shows that TV infections may assist the transmission of HIV-1 (Cohen, 1997).

Although the World Health Organisation (WHO) estimated that there were 10 million new cases of TV in Western Europe in 1996, in England the incidence of new cases has declined. In 1985 there were 14,304 new cases. This dropped to 5237 by 1995 (Department of Health, 1996). This decline has been attributed to contact tracing, treatment of asymptomatic male partners and higher sanitation standards (Mohanty, 1990). It is important to note, however, that the figures do not include those individuals who are asymptomatic or carriers of infection, or those who seek treatment outside genito-urinary medicine (GUM) clinics (DoH, 1996).

Trichomonas vaginalis is a flagellated protozoan that causes a sexually transmitted infection. It lives as a parasite which causes disease in the genital tract. It chiefly affects women, and adheres itself to the mucous membranes of the vagina (Rein and Muller, 1990). It can also effect the urethra, although this is less common. Apart from TV, there are two other species of trichomoniasis that are site specific: *Trichomonas tenax*, which lives in the mouth, and *Pentatrichomonas hominis*, which is found in the large intestine and is often associated with diarrhoea.

Treatment for TV is inexpensive and effective. However, resistance to the curative drug metronidazole is on the increase (Barat and Bloland, 1997; Petrin et al, 1998). Hence, research into alternative antibiotics and strategies to manage patients with drug resistance to TV is necessary. In addition, many cases of TV in men are not picked up. This is because it is often asymptomatic, it is difficult to diagnose and symptoms are often too minor to prompt a visit to the GUM clinic. Thus, men can be reservoirs of infection harbouring the parasite in the urethra (Holmes, 1990). Consequently, where partners of infected women are not treated, re-infection is common.

EPIDEMIOLOGY

Sexual contact, via vaginal and seminal fluid, is by far the most predominant form of transmission of TV between male–female partners. *Trichomonas vaginalis* can live for several hours in body fluids outside the body. Potentially, it could be transmitted through these body fluids, or by objects and materials that retain vaginal or seminal fluid, such as sponges and towels. However, there is no documented evidence to elucidate this (Rein and Muller, 1990). There also appears to be no published evidence on the transmission of TV among men who have sex with men, or women who have sex with women.

Five per cent of babies born to infected mothers will acquire TV in the birth canal. In these cases, the genito-urinary tract of the baby is affected. If the baby is treated with the same antibiotics given to adult patients, this infection poses no known risk. Nevertheless, it is not clear whether having TV during pregnancy has any adverse effects on pregnancy outcomes (Gulmezoglu, 1996a).

Trichomonas vaginalis will often be diagnosed with a concurrent STI or genital tract infection. For example, 20% of cases are diagnosed in association with gonorrhoea, 10% in association with candida and 5% in association with non-specific genital infections (Adler, 1995). It is recommended, therefore, to give a routine screen for all STIs and genital infections where TV is suspected.

It is difficult to obtain accurate statistics and information on the prevalence levels of TV. Estimates can be made based on figures from GUM clinics, GPs, family planning clinics, gynaecology services and other relevant sources. Establishing an accurate picture is even harder in developing countries due to poor availability of statistics and the lack of regular epidemiological surveys (Osujih, 1997). This sketchy picture inhibits the effective direction of resources and management and control of TV infection.

SIGNS AND SYMPTOMS

Symptoms for TV infection mimic other STIs, complicated by the concurrent diagnosis of TV with other genito-urinary tract infections. Hence, it is less easy to attribute the signs presented to TV.

Up to 75% of women with TV are symptomatic. Women will most frequently present with a combination of the following symptoms:

- an excessive vaginal discharge;

- a green-yellow vaginal discharge;

- vulvo-vaginal soreness and itching.

In addition, though less common, women may present with further symptoms:

- an offensive smelling discharge;

- dysparaeunia;

- dysuria;

- lower abdominal discomfort.

The parasite can be detected in vaginal secretions, in the urethra, in the Bartholin's gland and in the Skene's gland (Gulmezoglu, 1996a).

Women have an estimated three to 28-day incubation period, yet this is not always clear as many women notice the first symptoms of TV during or immediately after a menstrual period (Catterall, 1972).

Trichomonas vaginalis infection in women, that presents in isolation of other STIs, does not cause serious complications such as ectopic pregnancy and infertility, which are associated with gonorrhoea and chlamydia. Hence, the prime concerns of women suffering from TV infection are:

- the discomfort and inconvenience of the pruritus and the discharge (often exacerbated during menstruation);

- the time off work required;

▶ the psychological impact of the symptoms and the diagnosis.

The majority of men with trichomonal infection are asymptomatic. Thus, they have no distinct symptoms of the infected prostate gland, urethra or seminal vesicles (Osujih, 1997). It is also difficult to detect TV in males if the their last sexual contact with an infected partner was more than 48 hours prior to the examination. Hence, the symptoms of TV are hard to diagnose and differentiate from symptoms of other STIs. Nevertheless, men carry the parasite and transmit it sexually. Those men who do present as symptomatic, or as a sexual contact of TV, may present with any combination of the following symptoms:

▶ discharge from the penis;

▶ dysuria or frequency;

▶ testicular pain or tenderness;

▶ lower abdominal pain.

Trichomonas vaginalis is a well-established cause of non-gonococcal urethritis (NGU) in men (Rein and Muller, 1990). However, TV is invariably confirmed when NGU responds to metronidazole after it has not responded to other treatment already given.

EXAMINATION, DIAGNOSIS AND TESTS

A careful medical and sexual history should be taken before any physical examination is made. A high-risk profile for TV would be similar to those of any STI, namely:

▶ a change in sexual partner;

▶ multiple sexual partners;

▶ recurrent symptoms;

▶ symptoms in a partner;

▶ general symptoms – abdominal pain, dysuria, dyspareunia, menstrual problems (Davis, 1998).

The physical examination should be comprehensive. For women, an external examination is necessary of the vulva, pubic hair, surrounding skin and the perianal area. In addition, a digital examination of the vagina should be conducted.

On external examination, signs of TV would be inflammation and erythema of the vulva. Equally, a discharge may be visible on the vulva before a speculum is introduced.

The internal vaginal examination would include passing the speculum to visualise the cervix, the posterior and anterior fornix, and the vaginal walls. A vaginal pH should be recorded with litmus paper. Swabs should be taken from the vaginal walls, the cervix and the posterior fornix to screen for concurrent STIs. It is the latter swab which would be used to detect TV. A frothy yellow discharge is indicative of TV. The vaginal walls may appear inflamed and erythematous. In addition, a strawberry red cervix, not easily observed by the naked eye, but which may be visualised by colposcopy, will also indicate TV (Lossick, 1982).

For men, an examination would include an external examination of the scrotum, pubic hair, surrounding skin, perianal area, penis and urethra. Swabs should be taken from the urethra and a two-glass urine sample. This is to eliminate concurrent STIs. In most GUM clinics TV is not specifically tested for in men unless indicated by contact with a sexual partner with the infection.

TESTING

Various methods are available for the diagnosis of TV infection. The most common method is a wet preparation slide for microscopy. A sample of vaginal or urethral fluid should be obtained from the posterior fornix in women and from the urethra in men. The sample should then be added to the saline on the slide. A cover slip is put over the mixture. This is examined under the microscope. *Trichomonas vaginalis* is recognised clearly by the jerky movements of the protozoa flagella. TV organisms are detected in 40–80% of cases. The sensitivity of the test depends on the number of parasites in the vaginal or urethral sample and the competence of the examiner.

Samples from the aforementioned sites can be added to a culture medium. *Trichomonas vaginalis* is detected in the laboratory. Recent research has demonstrated the efficacy of In-Pouch TV culture as twice as effective as wet mount microscopy. Ohlemeyer et al (1998) have suggested that this is a good test for TV because of its long shelf-life, relatively low expense, and high sensitivity.

Trichomonas vaginalis is also often reported on Papanicolaou (Pap) smears from the cervix. The Pap smear has a sensitivity of about 60–70% (Lossick, 1982). However, it is hard to identify TV on a Pap smear, so this may lead to a large number of false positives (Rein and Muller, 1990).

TREATMENT

Metronidazole and the group of nitroimidazole drugs have been the treatment of choice for the past 30 years. Metronidazole is administered over five days or as a stat dose. It is advised that the antibiotic is taken with food and that the patient avoids alcohol. This is because, taken with metronidazole, alcohol may cause nausea, vomiting, abdominal pain and headache (British Medical Association, 1994). Trials have demonstrated that side effects are more common when the stat doses are administered rather than the five-day course (Gulmezoglu, 1996b). Repeat testing is recommended at one week and thirty days if treatment failure is suspected.

Equivalent topical creams and gels have demonstrated efficacy in relief of symptoms, not as a parasitological cure (Gulmezoglu, 1996b).

Treating people who have an allergy or a resistance to metronidazole is a challenge. However, promising results with the use of paromomycin cream have been shown (Coelho, 1997; Nyirjesy et al, 1998).

CONCLUSION

With the new evidence suggesting an association between TV infection and ease of HIV-1 transmission, we need to re-focus our attention on this lesser known STI. Hence, research needs to develop in the following main areas: the pathogenesis of TV, testing and treatment. Such developments should improve the management and control of TV.

Furthermore, the results of the research need to be cascaded more widely among the disciplines of gynaecology, family planning, GUM and general practice. Such an approach should encourage collaboration so that care can be improved, the incidence of TV can be reduced further and resources for TV can be directed appropriately (Petrin et al, 1998; Waghorn et al, 1998).

Case study

Tara visited her local GP complaining of a yellow and smelly discharge. She also had an itchy and sore vagina. Tara explained that this change had begun four days previously, towards the end of her menstrual period.

She had last had sexual intercourse two weeks earlier with her regular partner of three years. She used the contraceptive pill and she said she had used condoms when she had had sex outside the relationship. Her main concern was the discomfort the symptoms caused her, but she was also embarrassed to have sex with her partner, who had commented that he found her discharge smelly and offensive.

The GP suggested that a genito-urinary medicine clinic would offer a faster and more comprehensive service. Tara attended her local GUM clinic with a referral letter. Following a similar assessment, the doctor suggested that Tara should have a routine screen, which included a variety of tests to investigate for sexually transmitted and genital infections. The tests included internal and external examination of the genitals, blood tests and a digital examination of the vagina.

Tara was diagnosed with *Trichomonas vaginalis* and bacterial vaginosis. The doctor explained that the TV would account for the tenderness Tara experienced during examination and the discharge. She was assured that the smell was a typical symptom of bacterial vaginosis, and was given a five-day course of metronidazole.

Tara had a more detailed discussion with the health adviser about her diagnosis and its implications. Tara said that she was pleased to have some treatment that would make her feel comfortable again. However, she was concerned that her partner, who did not seem to have symptoms would be reluctant to attend the clinic. She affirmed that she would not have difficulty abstaining from sexual intercourse until the treatment was completed.

Tara's partner did attend. He was diagnosed with non-gonococcal urethritis (NGU) and given the same antibiotics. Tara and her partner attended the clinic for repeat tests and were both found clear of infection and of concurrent STIs.

References

Adler, M.W. (1995) *ABC of Sexually Transmitted Diseases*. London: BMJ Publishing Group.

Barat, L.M., Bloland, P.B. (1997) Drug resistance among malaria and other parasites. *Infectious Disease Clinics of North America*; 11: 4, 969–987.

British Medical Association (1994) *The New Guide to Medicines and Drugs*. London: Dorling Kindersley.

Caterall, R.D. (1972) Trichomonal infection of the genital tract. *Medical Clinics of North America*; 56, 1203.

Cohen, M.S. , Hoffman, I.F., Royce, R.A., et al. (1997) Reduction of concentration of HIV-1 in semen after treatment of urethritis: implications for prevention of sexual transmission of HIV-1. *The Lancet*; 349: 9096, 1868–1873.

Coelho, D.D. (1997) Metronidazole-resistant trichomoniasis successfully treated with paromomycin. *Genito-urinary Medicine*; 73: 5, 397–398.

Davis, A. (1998) Chlamydia: the most common sexually transmitted disease infection. *Nursing Times*; 94: 5, 56–58.

Department of Health (1996) *Sexually transmitted diseases, England 1995; new cases seen at NHS genito-urinary medicine clinics*. London: DoH.

Gulmezoglu, A.M. (1996a) Trichomoniasis treatment during pregnancy. In Neilson, J.P. et al (eds) *Pregnancy and Childbirth Module of the Cochrane Database of Systematic Reviews*. The Cochrane Library. The Cochrane Collaboration; issue 1. Oxford: Update Software.

Gulmezoglu, A.M. (1996b) Trichomoniasis treatment in women. In Garner, P. et al (eds) *Infectious Diseases Module of the Cochrane Database of Systematic Reviews*. The Cochrane Library. The Cochrane Collaboration; issue 1. Oxford: Update Software.

Holmes, K.K. (1990) *Sexually Transmitted Diseases*. London: McGraw-Hill.

Lossick, J.G. (1982) Treatment of *Trichomonas vaginalis* infections. *Review of Infectious Diseases*; 4: 4, 801.

Mohanty, K.C. (1990) Trichomoniasis. *British Journal of Sexual Medicine*; 17: 4, 210–12.

Nyirjesy, P., Sobel, J.D., Weitz, et al. (1998) Difficult to treat trichomoniasis: results with paromomycin cream. *Clinical Infectious Diseases*; 26: 4, 986–988.

Ohlemeyer, C.L., Hornberger, L.L., Lynch, D.A. et al (1998) Diagnosis of *Trichomonas vaginalis* in adolescent females: In-Pouch TV culture versus wet-mount microscopy. *Journal of Adolescent Health*. 22: 3, 205–208.

Osujih, M. (1997) The 'other' sexually transmitted diseases: a case for public health education. *Journal of the Royal Society of Health*; 117: 6, 351–354.

Petrin, D., Delgaty, K., Bhatt, R. et al (1998) Clinical and microbiological aspects of *Trichomonas vaginalis*. *Clinical Microbiology Review*; 11: 2, 300–317.

Rein, M.F. and Muller, M. (1990) *Trichomonas vaginalis* and trichomaniasis. In Holmes, K.K. et al (eds) *Sexually Transmitted Diseases*. London: McGraw-Hill.

Waghorn, D.J., Tucker, P.K., Chia, Y. et al (1998) Collaborative approach to improve the detection and management of trichomoniasis in a low prevalence district. *International Journal of STDs and AIDS*; 9: 3, 164–7.

11. Parasitic infections

Marsh Gelbart

INTRODUCTION

Sexually acquired ectoparasites, creatures that can live in or on the skin, are universally loathed. The prospect of interlopers, moving and feeding amongst your genitalia, is enough to bring a shudder to any individual. Nevertheless, when examined close up, ectoparasites are fascinating examples of design superbly evolved to purpose.

There are two main perpetrators of genital infestations: scabies mites and pubic lice. They are normally considered to be mere nuisances, but their physical and psychological impact is out of all proportion to their diminutive size. Symptoms of infestation usually include itching, erythema, irritation and inflammation. Scratching the burrows and lesions associated with mites and lice can lead to minor but unpleasant bacterial infections of the skin. The emotional consequences of catching an ectoparasite can be considerable. They are wrongly associated in the public mind with 'loose morals' and lack of sexual hygiene. In addition, they can be seen as visible stigmata of unfaithfulness.

SCABIES MITES

Scabies is an infestation found on a world-wide basis. It is caused by *Sarcoptes scabiei*. This burrowing creature is an arachnid, having four pairs of legs. As an obligate parasite, it cannot live for long on the human body (Marks, 1997). The mite is approximately 0.4mm in length, and when examined at anything over 40× magnification, it looks like a cross between a spiny tortoise and some mythical prehistoric animal.

The male scabies mite lives simply to fertilise the female and then dies; the larger female lives on. It uses its powerful front two pairs of legs, the final joints of which have suckers and cutting edges, to carve a burrow for itself in the stratum corneum. These burrows are more visible than the mite – they vary from 1–4mm in length and are a greyish-white in appearance. Within its den, the mite lays between 10 and 25 eggs, and deposits its body wastes. The mite tunnels at an approximate rate of 2mm a day, just beneath the surface of the skin. After fulfilling its function as a breeding machine, the mite dies inside the burrow. The eggs take three or four days to hatch. The larvae scrabble their way to the surface where they dig moulting pouches. There, the larvae transform into their adult form and the cycle recommences.

The scabies mite was identified as early as 1687 (Wistreich, 1992), but its mode of transmission was not well understood. Much of our knowledge of the scabies mite and how transmittable it is, comes from a series of eccentric experiments carried out in the 1940s. The research was based at Fairholme House on the outskirts of Sheffield (Andrews, 1978).

The authorities of the period were worried about potential epidemics of scabies in crowded barracks and air-raid shelters. Contemporary theories held that scabies was a particularly easily transmittable complaint. To test the validity of this theory, a group of conscientious objectors volunteered to be deliberately exposed to scabies. The intention was to assess modes of transmission. The unwashed blankets and underwear of soldiers infested with scabies were given to the volunteers. They slept naked under the former and wore the latter – heroically – for a week at a time. Despite this exposure to potential infestation, the volunteers didn't develop scabies. Only after volunteers shared the beds of soldiers with scabies did they catch the mite. The Fairholme experiment demonstrated that the scabies mite is not readily transmittable through contact with inanimate objects – only after prolonged skin contact with an infected individual is the mite likely to be transmitted. Although sexual contact is the main mode of transmission amongst adults, poverty and overcrowding (sharing beds) are other factors implicated.

Signs, symptoms and treatment

The primary symptom of scabies is an intense itching sensation, often worse at night. The itching doesn't usually start until the infected individual becomes sensitised. This can take up to a month after the mites have commenced tunnelling. If a person has been previously sensitised, a subsequent infection leads to a much swifter onset of symptoms. The affected area is usually symmetrical and is characterised by an eczematous rash, often criss-crossed by scratch marks. These self-inflicted scratches can hide the burrows themselves. As well as the genitalia and lower abdomen, the mites are classically found on the flexor aspects of the wrists, and between the finger webs. Other areas affected are the palms, armpits and buttocks, the knee, elbow, ankle and around the aureole of the nipple. The head and neck of adults, but not children, are usually unaffected by scabies mites, unless the infested adult has an impaired immune system.

The normal colony of scabies mites on an affected individual numbers from 10 to 50. The body's immune response leads to scratching, which helps limit the number of mites. If a person has an impaired immune response through age, illness, or chemical suppression of the immune system, then the sum total of mites may reach into the millions. In this case, the skin has extensive crusted lesions holding vast quantities of the mite. The condition is known as Norwegian scabies or, more accurately, as crusted scabies. Crusted scabies is particularly infectious; it is responsible for frequent non-sexual transmission in hospital wards and other institutions.

It can be surprisingly difficult to diagnose scabies. It is often misdiagnosed as atopic dermatitis. The burrows are difficult to identify, and standard microscopic examination of skin scrapings doesn't always reveal the mite. The technique of epiluminescence microscopy allows a more detailed study of the skin and a better chance of discovering mites (Argenziano et al, 1997).

Treatment options have, until recently, focused around topical applications (Table 1). Topical applications can be time consuming and difficult to apply. Several cases of crusted scabies have recently been successfully treated by a single oral dose of invermectin (Aubin, 1995; Burkhart, 1997). Whatever the chosen treatment option, the index patient, his or her sexual contacts and members of the household will all need treatment. As protein from the dead mites and their faecal waste continues to trigger an immune response, itching can continue for several weeks. It needs to be made clear to patients that this may be the case, otherwise people with scabies often return to their doctor or clinic requesting retreatment for persistent symptoms. Calamine lotion may be helpful in alleviating itching. Practitioners should avoid the automatic assumption of reinfestation and unnecessary retreatment.

Table 1. Two representative treatment regimes for scabies

▸ **Regime 1** Lyclear (permethrin 5% dermal cream). Apply to whole of body below the neck. Wash off after 8–24 hours.

▸ **Regime 2** Quellada (lindane 1% in a lotion base). Apply to whole of body below the neck. Wash off after 24 hours. Should not be used on pregnant women or young children.

PUBIC LICE

The pubic louse, *Phthirus pubis,* resembles the head louse, but it is somewhat flatter and broader with a crab-like appearance, hence its alternative name of crab louse. It is about 2mm in diameter, and brownish in colour. The pubic louse has three pairs of legs. Its bottom two pairs are equipped with heavy-duty, curved claws, designed to grip the coarser body hairs. The pubic louse and the scabies mite were initially confused, the opinion being that they were different stages of the life-cycle of the same pest. The pubic louse was first described by Linnaeus in 1758 (Andrews, 1978). Although not as common as the head louse, the pubic louse is now far more common than body lice, which have declined with the advent of easy laundering and ironing of clothing. Fortunately, the pubic louse, unlike its closely related cousin the body louse, does not carry fatal diseases such as typhus.

Pubic lice can be found all over the world. They affect people of all classes and socio-economic backgrounds. One academic paper contends that pubic lice infestations are more likely to be found in people with a low socio-economic status (Gilles et al, 1991). Amongst the sexually active aged between 15 and 19 they are more commonly found in females. Over the age of 20, males are more likely to have crabs (Wistreich, 1992). An infestation with pubic lice often runs concurrently with other sexual infections. As always, any person attending a genito-urinary medicine

(GUM) clinic should have a general screen for other sexually transmitted infections (STIs).

The pubic louse favours the hair around the genitals, but can also occasionally be found in the armpits, facial hair, eyebrows and eyelashes. While phthiriasis, or pubic louse infestation is normally spread through sexual contact, it can be passed on through contact with infected bedding, towels and from pubic hairs left loose on toilet seats. This is because – unlike the scabies mite – the pubic louse can remain viable and active for several hours off the body.

Signs, symptoms and treatment

Itching is the primary symptom of pubic lice. Although well camouflaged, pubic lice can be discerned with the help of a magnifying glass. In addition, the lice lay their eggs at the base of coarse body hair where they can sometimes be seen with the naked eye. The chitinous envelope cemented to the base of the hair is known as a nit. It takes about a week for the nit to hatch, and approximately another week for the larva to mature into a fully fledged louse (Nicol Thin, 1982). After clambering down a pubic hair, the louse feeds from its unfortunate host approximately a dozen times a day. After feeding, the crab louse swells and excretes a reddish excrement. If infestation is heavy, characteristic sky-blue spots can be observed in the infested areas. These spots are the marks caused by tiny haemorrhages – they will disperse after a few days. It is rare that an infestation goes much beyond ten adult pubic lice.

Topical applications are the usual course of treatment (Table 2). Permethrin preparations have taken over from lindane as the treatment of choice since 1996, as there has been some concern over adverse central nervous system reactions with the latter medication (Downs, 1997). Treatment regimes for lice need to be rotated, as the insects develop resistance. Clothing should be washed on a hot cycle.

Table 2. Two representative treatment regimes for pubic lice

▶ **Regime I** Prioderm (malathion 1% in a shampoo base). Apply to pubic areas and body hair other than scalp. Leave on for five minutes, rinse and repeat after three days.

> ▸ **Regime 2** Lyclear (permethrin 1%, cream rinse in an alcohol base). Apply to pubic areas and body hair other than scalp. Leave on for 10 minutes, rinse and dry.

One of the problems that occurs in the treatment of pubic lice, is the tendency to self-treat, because people are often too ashamed to attend their family doctor or a GUM clinic. While appropriate shampoos or applications can be bought over the counter at a pharmacist, people can be too embarrassed to ask for advice. As a result, highly dubious 'cures' can be attempted. The author has come across one young man who attended clinic after using lighter fluid to burn off his pubic hair. The lice had been burned off, but so had much of the patient's skin!

CONCLUSION

Infestation by ectoparasites is a relatively common and distressing condition. Infestation rates are a reminder that the parasites are well evolved to exist within their specific ecological niche. While the means of eradicating sexually transmitted infestations are readily available, their application is hindered by social attitudes and ignorance.

Case study 1

Sixteen-year-old Ian recently attended a local genito-urinary medicine (GUM) clinic. For the last five days Ian's genital area had felt itchy. He had scratched and chafed the area about his pubic hair and as a consequence it was excoriated and sore.

One of the clinic doctors had to frequently reassure Ian about confidentiality in GUM clinics before he was able to obtain a sexual history from the patient. It was eventually ascertained that Ian was heterosexual, and had enjoyed his first episode of intercourse some six days previously. He had no urethral discharge or other signs of additional sexual infection.

Although reluctant to consent to a physical examination, Ian eventually agreed. The importance of screening for a range of other sexually transmitted infections was explained. Again, he was averse to having any swabs taken from his urethra, having heard 'horror stories' from older friends. Only after much reassurance, and a discussion of the importance of screening, did he consent.

During physical examination, several nits could be seen cemented close to the base of a number of Ian's pubic hairs. A nurse was able to find several lice hidden amongst the hair. One of the lice was removed for examination by microscope to confirm the diagnosis. After careful examination of the genitalia, no scabies burrows were found – it is possible to have the two infestations running concurrently. Nor was anything of note discovered on microscopic examination of the swabs taken from Ian's urethra – when culture results returned from the hospital laboratory some days later, all were negative.

After receiving a diagnosis of pubic lice, and an assurance that the Prioderm shampoo provided would rapidly eradicate his unwanted guests, Ian relaxed considerably. He agreed to have a chat with one of the clinic's health advisers, who confirmed that Ian had only ever had the one sexual partner. He had slept with this partner on only one occasion, after meeting her at a party. All Ian knew of her was her first name. Although it was extremely unlikely that he would see her again, Ian promised to discuss his infestation with her, should they ever meet. He declined a contact slip. The health adviser verified that Ian understood what pubic lice were and knew how to apply the medication he had been given. A basic discussion on sexual health and condom usage took place. The health adviser checked that Ian knew how to apply a condom correctly. Ian left the clinic in a much happier frame of mind than he entered with.

Case study 2

Norman, a 32-year-old married man who attended a GUM clinic some forty miles from his home town, had been in a previously monogamous marriage for the last seven years. Some six weeks previously, he had had unprotected penetrative sex with a casual female partner he had met while away on a course. For the last two weeks, Norman had been suffering from an intense itching sensation around his genitals and lower abdomen. The itching was worse at night. Norman attended clinic on the assumption that he had picked up a sexual illness. He believed that 'he may have caught something' from his casual partner.

Norman saw one of the clinic's doctors and agreed to have a full sexual health screen (an HIV test was offered but declined as he was still within the window period of twelve weeks). On examination, no evidence of pubic lice could be found. However, there were several tiny tracks, some three to four millimetres long at the top of his scrotal sac. Norman had scratched heavily around the itchy areas. The skin around his groin was torn and damaged, making a firm diagnosis even more difficult. However, the doctor noted more suspicious burrows in the finger webs of both hands. This led to a presumptive diagnosis of scabies mites.

Direct microscopy didn't show any unequivocal evidence of any other sexually transmitted infection. Norman denied having any penile discharge, but the slide made from his urethral swab showed a large number of pus cells. An epidemiological diagnosis of non-specific urethritis (NSU) was made. Norman was given sufficient permethrin 5% dermal cream to apply to himself, his wife and his two small children. Staff checked that Norman knew how to apply the lotion. In addition, a course of oxytetracycline tablets was given to treat the NSU. Norman had twice had unprotected intercourse with his wife since sleeping with his casual partner. Norman was having real difficulties coping with his diagnosis, so he was asked to have a chat with one of the health advisers.

The health adviser ascertained that Norman was horrified that his wife and children would also require treatment with permethrin. He was also mortified that his wife would need to attend a clinic for investigations and treatment of NSU. Norman was terribly concerned that his relationship with his wife may collapse. After much careful discussion, Norman agreed to tell his wife about his attendance at the clinic and the reason for it. Norman agreed to take a contact slip to give to his wife with his diagnoses (his casual partner could not be contacted). He understood the need to avoid intercourse until he and his wife had completed their treatment for NSU and had tests of cure.

The patient did not attend our clinic again, but a telephone call was received some weeks later from a health adviser based at a GUM clinic in Norman's home town. Norman's wife had attended for treatment of NSU and for follow-up for itching, post-treatment from scabies. It is not known how severely damaged the relationship between Norman and his wife had become.

References

Andrews, M. (1978) *The life that lives on man.* London: Arrow Books.

Argenziano, G., Fabbrocini, G., Delfino, M. (1997) Eluminescence microscopy: a new approach to in vivo detection of *Sarcoptes scabiei. Archives of Dermatology;* 133: 6, 751–753.

Aubin, F. (1995) Ivermectin for crusted (Norwegian) scabies. *The New England Journal of Medicine;* 332: 9, 612.

Burkhart, K.M., Burkhart, C.N., Burkhart, C.G. (1997) Comparing topical scabietic treatments will soon become extinct. *Archives of Dermatology;* 133: 10, 1314.

Downs, A. (1997) Comparing antiscabies treatments. *Archives of Dermatology;* 133: 4, 526.

Gilles, D., Slepon, R., Karsenty, E. et al (1990) Socio-demographic factors associated with *Pediculosis capitis* and *pubis* among young adults in the Israeli Defense Forces. *Public Health Review;* 18: 4, 345–350.

Marks, R. (1997) *Roxburgh's Common Skin Diseases.* London: Chapman and Hall Medical.

Nicol Thin, R. (1982) *Lecture Notes on Sexually Transmitted Diseases.* London: Blackwell Scientific Publications.

Wistreich, G.A. (1992) *The Sexually Transmitted Diseases: A Current Approach.* East Los Angeles College: WCB Group.

12. Sexually spread hepatitis

Caroline Smales

INTRODUCTION

Hepatitis literally means inflammation of the liver, but the spectrum of disease can range from subclinical, in the majority of cases, detectable only by abnormal liver enzymes, if at all, to fulminant hepatitis, chronic hepatitis, liver cancer and, ultimately, to premature death (Zuckerman, 1997a). Viruses are the most significant cause of hepatitis, but it may also be caused by excessive alcohol, drugs, chemicals and other types of infectious disease.

Viral hepatitis is caused by a unique group of viruses that only have an affinity for the liver and are classified alphabetically, currently ranging from A to G.

There is evidence of viruses beyond G, but these have yet to be clearly identified and their clinical implications evaluated. Hepatitis A and E (HAV and HEV) tend to cause acute hepatitis (with a duration of less than six months), Hepatitis B, C, D and G (HBV, HCV, HDV, HGV) can cause both acute and chronic hepatitis (with a duration of more than six months) (British Liver Trust, 1996).

THE SIGNIFICANCE OF THESE VIRUSES

All these viruses can be transmitted from person to person by more than one route. The major routes of transmission are either via the faecal–oral route in the case of hepatitis A and E, and via the blood-borne route in hepatitis B, C, D and G. However, depending on the sexual activities practised and the frequency of sexual intimacy all have the potential to be sexually transmitted, in fact, one-third of cases of HBV are spread in this way (Gurevich, 1993).

The Hep Risk Advisory Board (1996) has found that knowledge regarding this risk is generally poor and people are unknowingly putting themselves at risk. Therefore, health care professionals must be aware, for their own health as well as for the health of others, that hepatitis can cause serious health problems and may be sexually spread and, in particular, that unlike some other sexually transmitted infections (STIs), such as gonorrhoea, syphilis and chlamydia, it cannot be treated with antibiotics. However, HAV, HBV and HDV can be prevented through vaccination, and the risk from all the other forms can be reduced by safer sexual practices.

Although, in the majority of cases, people recover from hepatitis with no sequelae, they can become carriers of HBV, HCV, HDV and possibly HGV, and have a greater chance of developing chronic forms of liver disease which, at best, may cause a continuous feeling of malaise, and at worst may cause cirrhosis, liver cancer and ultimately a premature death (Carlisle, 1997). This risk is particularly high if HBV infection is spread to babies at the time of their birth (Smith et al, 1994; Zuckerman, 1997b).

The Department of Health guidelines recommend that, for their own protection, unless infected health care workers can demonstrate sufficient antibody protection to HBV, they may not work in high-risk areas such as invasive surgery (DoH, 1993). In addition, HBV-antigen-positive health care workers can be restricted in the type of work they do as they must not be involved in exposure-prone procedures (EPP) because of the risk of their blood contaminating a patient's open tissues (DoH, 1993).

Regardless of the viral cause, the acute symptoms of hepatitis are indistinguishable: malaise, anorexia, mild abdominal pain and fever, and arthralgia. However, there are some important epidemiological differences.

ENTERIC INFECTIOUS HEPATITIS

HAV and HEV mainly cause acute hepatitis and only rarely a chronic form. They are both found worldwide and are spread via ingestion of water (and/or food) contaminated with infected faecal material.

Some 1290 cases of HAV were reported to the Public Health Laboratory Service (PHLS) in 1997, with the number of reported cases having fallen in the last six to seven years. HEV has been responsible for very large water-borne outbreaks in Asia, and North and East Africa, but cases reported to the PHLS in the UK were 13 in 1994, rising to only 22 reports in 1997.

HAV more commonly affects young children, with the majority of cases subclinical or mild, but resulting in lifetime immunity. Infected adults tend to have a more severe or prolonged illness which is sometimes accompanied by fulminant hepatitis. However, in the main it is followed by complete recovery and lifelong immunity.

In contrast, HEV affects mainly young adults and does not seem to confer good immunity, so reinfection is possible (Goldsmith et al, 1992).

There is no carrier state with either HAV or HEV and currently there is no evidence that either can be spread to the unborn foetus. HEV appears to have a much lower rate of secondary spread – about 2%, which is presumed to be due to its lability (chemical instability) – compared with 15% observed with HAV (Skidmore, 1995).

The incubation period for both ranges from two to six weeks, although HEV may extend to nine weeks and diagnosis is made serologically by the detection of HAV- or HEV-specific antibody. Treatment for both is conservative. Overall mortality for HAV and HEV is about 0.1% in the young to 1% in adults. Pregnant women, however, seem to be exceptionally susceptible to HEV and mortality is reported to be as high as 20% (Skidmore, 1995).

There is evidence that people with chronic HCV have a higher incidence of dying if they become infected with HAV (Vento, 1998). Currently HAV vaccination is recommended by the Department of Health (1996) for certain groups (Table 1).

Table I. Groups recommended to have hepatitis A vaccine:

- Travellers to endemic areas
- Military workers
- Workers in child care centres
- Homosexual men
- Sanitation workers
- Anyone with chronic hepatitis C

BLOOD-BORNE VIRUSES CAUSING HEPATITIS

Overall the incidence of HBV, HCV, HDV and HGV is low in England and Wales compared with the rest of the world. However, if people travel to other countries there is an increased risk of exposure.

The hepatitis B virus

Hepatitis B has a long incubation period of between six weeks and six months. The World Health Organisation (WHO) estimates that 350 million people worldwide are infected, and that it is killing one million people every year (British Liver Trust, 1996).

In England and Wales approximately 600 acute cases of HBV are reported to the PHLS each year and there are thought to be 50,000 chronic carriers. The prevalence in the general population of England and Wales is 0.5%, and 5% in homosexual men, while in South-East Asia and sub-Saharan Africa it is as high as 30% (Boag, 1991).

Acute hepatitis ranges from subclinical to fulminant hepatic failure in 2% of cases. Fortunately, 90–95% of acute cases make a full recovery with no sequelae and conferred lifelong immunity. Unfortunately, in around 5–10% of cases the immune system does not completely clear the virus and people may become chronically infected carriers facing the possibility of chronic liver problems. The majority (60%) of HBV cases are subclinical, detectable only by serological tests. However, others (40%) will have acute symptoms of hepatitis (Hart, 1990).

Predominantly a blood-borne virus, routes of transmission include vertical – from mother to baby – and horizontal – via any activity that allows the transfer of infected blood, for instance in the presence of poor sterilising techniques through surgical instruments (e.g. tattooing and ear piercing), and where there is poor screening through blood transfusion and organ donation, as well as sharing needles, toothbrushes and razors. The virus is also detected in other body fluids such as saliva, semen and vaginal fluid, and it can be spread via sexual intercourse (Davison et al, 1987).

Diagnosis of HBV is made serologically. It has three antigens in its structure that can evoke the production of three corresponding antibodies (Table 2). Failure of the immune system to produce corresponding antibodies results in the sequelae already mentioned.

The detection of HBsAg (hepatitis B surface antigen) indicates current or chronic infection or a carrier state. The presence of HBeAg (hepatitis E antigen) points to viral replication or active infection being present in the acute phase, and this persists if the infection becomes chronic.

Anti-HBe antibodies signal viral suppression or clearance, while detection of anti-HBsAg equivalent shows that the patient has cleared the virus indicating recovery. Another possible antigen is HBcAg, although this stays within the liver and is not detectable in the blood; however, antibodies to HBcAg are an indicator of recent or current infection.

Table 2. HBV antigens and corresponding antibodies

Antigen markers

HBsAg – hepatitis B surface antigen (found in blood)

HBcAg – hepatitis B core antigen (found in liver only)

HBeAg – hepatitis B 'e' antigen (found in blood)

Antibody markers

Anti-HBsAg – antibody to hepatitis B surface antigen (found in blood)

Anti-HBcAg – antibody to hepatitis B core antigen (found in blood)

Anti-HBeAg – antibody to hepatitis B 'e' antigen (found in blood)

When an individual becomes a carrier there are two levels of infectivity indicated by blood tests, and people may have one or both:

▶ the presence of surface antigen, which is generally less serious;

▶ the presence of 'e' antigen signals a high level of viral replication in the blood and possibly other body fluids, resulting in a high risk of infecting others.

The hepatitis C virus

Hepatitis C is a worldwide health problem, and studies indicate that the virus is present in 0.2% of the UK population, with estimates that 450,000 people may be infected in the UK (British Liver Trust, 1996). In 1997, 2640 cases were reported to the PHLS in contrast with 241 reported cases in 1992. The incidence is higher in countries such as Japan, Italy and the Middle East, and is particularly prevalent in developing countries (Van der Poel et al, 1994). It was first identified in 1989, with routine antibody testing from 1991. It accounts for up to 90% of non-A, non-B hepatitis. It has an incubation period of six to eight weeks and can result in a carrier state in approximately 10% of cases (Group B, 1990).

HCV is thought to be less infectious than HBV, being primarily spread through blood transfusions, but it can be spread via needle sharing and also through vaginal and anal sexual activity. The risk of perinatal transmission is currently thought to be low. The majority of cases (90%) are clinically undetectable and more importantly, in contrast to HBV, 70–85% of acutely infected individuals progress to chronic active hepatitis (Alberti, 1992).

Once a person is chronically infected the virus is almost never cleared without treatment, and the history of chronic infection can vary dramatically. Some people will have clinically insignificant or minimal liver disease and never develop complications, the only evidence being by liver biopsy. Others have clinically apparent chronic hepatitis which may progress to liver damage slowly over 10–40 years. Ten to twenty per cent of chronic cases go on to develop cirrhosis within five to 30 years and will require a liver transplant, and approximately 10% will develop hepatocarcinoma (Benhamou, 1993). Currently there is no vaccine available for HCV, although research is ongoing.

The hepatitis D, F and G viruses

Hepatitis D requires the presence of HBV to replicate, and therefore infection can occur as a co-infection at the time of HBV acquisition, or as a superinfection of chronic HBV infection.

The presence of HDV appears to cause a more severe form of chronic hepatitis, with accelerated progression to complications of chronic hepatitis. Sexual and vertical transmission is less common than with HBV. Diagnosis is made serologically and treatment is conservative. Fortunately, the prevention of HDV can be afforded by HBV immunisation.

The designation of hepatitis F (HFV) is sometimes used to refer to an unidentified agent that possibly causes fulminant hepatitis (Deka et al, 1994).

Hepatitis G (HGV) was first identified in 1996 (Linnen et al, 1996). Transmission is primarily via blood and blood products, but it is also thought to be spread from infected mother to infant during childbirth. There is also some evidence for sexual transmission. It causes chronic infection, but the effects on sufferers' liver and health over time are unknown (Alter 1996; Lundberg 1997; Rubio et al 1997; Pujol et al, 1998).

SEXUAL TRANSMISSION

Sexual contact is an important means of transmission for viral hepatitis.

The ability of HAV to be transmitted to close personal contacts is explained by high concentrations of virus shed in faeces of infected people two weeks before the onset of symptoms (Shorey, 1982). Because many people are subclinically infected many are unaware that they are infectious.

HAV can be spread through anal and oral sex when the virus from faeces could inadvertently be ingested (Shorey, 1982). Although HEV is also shed in the faeces, there is no evidence that it may be transmitted through anal or oral sex.

The hepatitis B virus is 100 times more infectious than HIV (Ross and Dickerson, 1992). Even minute quantities of serum passing through tiny breaks in the skin and mucous membranes during vaginal and anal intercourse can lead to infection of sexual partners, with the risk even higher if a female partner is menstruating at the time. The virus can also be found in saliva, semen and vaginal fluids before and during the onset of acute and chronically infected cases, and during penetrative vaginal or anal sexual intercourse the virus may be transferred from the infected to the non-infected. As with all STIs the greater the number of partners the greater the chance of exposure and therefore the chance of infection. In 1997, out of the 624 reported cases of HBV to the PHLS, 54 were the result of sex between men and 83 were the result of heterosexual sex.

The extent to which HCV, HDV and HGV are spread sexually is still rather controversial. However, there is increasing evidence that HCV may also be spread very efficiently through vaginal and anal sexual intercourse, although a definitive study has not yet been done. Sexual transmission between monogamous couples is rare, but a study carried out at the Middlesex Hospital in 1991 demonstrated sexual transmission of HCV. This was linked to age, lifetime number of sexual partners, previous numbers of STIs, and HIV and HBV positivity (Tedder et al, 1991). Co-existing HIV infection may increase the efficiency of sexually transmitted HCV (Eyster et al, 1991).

Hepatitis G is a relatively newly discovered virus, but there is some evidence that it may also be spread sexually (Rubio et al, 1997). As yet there is no evidence of HDV being sexually transmitted.

It is important that in attempts to participate in safer alternatives to vaginal and anal sexual intercourse people do not also put themselves at risk. Mutual masturbation should not really pose a risk, but the transfer of viruses onto the hands could possibly allow them to spread into the body by ingestion (in the case of HAV) or through cuts and abrasions on the skin (in particular in the case of HBV).

Scarification and cutting practices for sexual pleasure or in sexual play should also be avoided. The risk of hepatitis transmission via oral sex is as yet unclear. However, some authors claim that HAV and HBV and possibly HCV can be spread via this route (Edwards and Carne, 1998). Again, the importance of oral sex as a method for the transmission of viruses may increase as other, higher risk sexual practices are avoided because of fear of acquiring HIV (Edwards and Carne, 1998).

PATHOLOGY, SIGNS AND SYMPTOMS

As has already been mentioned, symptoms of acute infection vary greatly in their severity and it is not unusual for their presence to go unnoticed. Whichever way these viruses enter the body they all have an affinity for the liver only, and once there cause inflammation and disruption of cellular (hepatocyte) function. Subsequent swelling of these liver cells leads to obstruction of bile flowing through the liver. This results in re-absorption of bile salts into the circulation, giving rise to many of the specific signs and symptoms of jaundice and itching. The reduction of bile being secreted into the gastrointestinal tract leads to pale faeces and dark urine.

Regardless of the type of virus, any acute symptoms will be similar and, in the majority of cases, are caused not by the virus but by the inflammation generated within the liver by the immune response (Table 3).

A small minority of people do not present with classic symptoms but present with arthralgia (pain in joints), arthritis (inflammation of the joints) and urticaria (skin rash with weals, and a small hard liver) – this is thought to be due to a vigorous immune response (antigen) to the virus and is associated with a poor prognosis.

Table 3. Symptom phases

Prodromal phase

Tends to be due to the viraemia and congestion in the liver. Symptoms:

► fatigue;

► anorexia and loss of desire to smoke (if previously a smoker);

► nausea/vomiting;

► flu-like symptoms (many people only ever have these symptoms);

► right upper quadrant pain (usually mild);

► altered bowel function – constipation/diarrhoea (25% of patients).

Icteric phase (classic phase)

Due to inflammatory process in the liver and obstruction of bile (25–35% of people get this). Symptoms:

► hepatomegaly;

► jaundice;

► dark urine and pale stool;

► pruritus (itching due to excess bile salts in the blood).

Convalescence phase

Symptoms:

► malaise;

► post-viral depression;

► urine/stool return to normal;

► liver returns to normal size.

LIVER FUNCTION TESTS

Three biochemical tests are characteristically elevated in viral hepatitis. Although these tests reflect the presence of damage or inflammation rather than measuring the function of the liver, they are used as a guide for the doctor in the diagnosis. They are:

► aminotransferases (transaminases) ALT and AST – enzymes released into blood in excess in liver cell necrosis 500 international units (iu)/L or greater (normal is 10–35iu/L);

▸ serum alkaline phosphatase – enzyme formed in bones/liver removed from blood by liver and excreted by bile (normal is 60–80mmol) is raised above normal;

▸ bilirubin – main bile pigment in humans normally found in small amounts in the blood (normal is 1–15mmol), but raised in hepatitis (to around 200iumol/L) causing yellow discoloration of skin (jaundice). It is not helpful in distinguishing between causes of liver disease, but reflects the liver's ability to take up, process and secrete bilirubin into the bile;

▸ prothrombin time is a test to assess blood clotting – this may be may be prolonged and is a good measure of liver malfunction.

TREATMENT

Treatment for acute viral hepatitis is conservative, involving observation and treatment of symptoms. However, in the case of chronic HBV and HCV there are two main approaches to treatment for patients who have had hepatitis for more than six months. This is:

▸ immunomodulation – alpha interferon is given to boost the individual's ability to use his or her own immune system. Unfortunately, this is only effective in less than 50% of cases of HBV, and 20% of HCV cases have a sustained response with complete eradication of the virus (Mangtani, 1995);

▸ antiviral agents – such as lamivudine, which appears to be effective in inhibiting viral replication in the case of HBV, and ribavirin in the case of HCV (Reichard, 1991).

In the case of liver failure a liver transplant may be the only option a patient has. The prognosis for this is generally quite good, in particular for those with chronic HBV, but not so good for those with chronic HCV – the liver in this instance appears to more readily become reinfected (Cowley and Webster, 1993).

PREVENTION

Unlike most other STIs, viral hepatitis cannot be treated and therefore prevention is vital. There are two main ways to prevent the sexual transmission of viral hepatitis: vaccination and a change in sexual behaviour.

Vaccination

HBV can be prevented by a genetically engineered and safe vaccine. The WHO wants to see universal immunisation for HBV to reduce deaths and carriers by 80% by the year 2001 (WHO, 1992).

As yet there is no vaccine currently available for HCV, although research is ongoing. Prevention of HDV is afforded by immunisation of HBV.

Immunisation can be given to people for prevention of HAV at GP and travel clinics; it is sometimes offered to homosexual men in GUM clinics. As yet there is no vaccine for HEV.

Safer sex

Although hepatitis viruses A to G have been identified, there are almost certainly others we have yet to identify, and their full clinical significance has yet to be realised, so change in sexual behaviour is vital.

The only way to completely avoid sexually transmitted hepatitis is to abstain from all sexual activities that involve the exchange of body fluids. A diagnosis of hepatitis can cause considerable anxiety and stress in people, usually relating to how they contracted the infection. It is therefore important that health care workers keep themselves well informed and are able to give factual, direct and non-judgmental sexual health advice.

Curtis et al (1995) suggest that safer sex means choosing sexual practices that carry less risk of STIs, HIV or unwanted pregnancy and that the aim for most people is to reduce risk to the level they consider acceptable.

CONCLUSION

Viral hepatitis is just one of the many infections that can be sexually transmitted. It can result in people becoming carriers of the virus and transmitting it to other sexual partners. It can range from a mild and self-limiting infection to chronic liver disease and premature death. However, unlike many other STIs it cannot be cured, but it can be prevented. In the case of HAV and HBV there is good safe protection in the form of vaccination; however, this must not lead to complacency as people must continue to be aware and engage in safer sexual practices in order to protect themselves from all forms of hepatitis as well as other STIs.

Case study

John, a 34-year-old, had been in a stable relationship with his girlfriend for a number of years. Recently he had casual unprotected vaginal intercourse with another woman. Four months later he was referred to the hospital by his GP with clinical signs of hepatitis: he was jaundiced, anorexic, nauseous and lethargic. Investigations found his LFTs were ten times the normal and he had positive markers for HBV. Further questioning revealed that John had no history of drug use, needle sharing or blood transfusions. In the following week John's condition deteriorated and he went into complete liver failure. He was immediately transferred to a specialist liver unit where the only treatment option for him was a liver transplant.

Before becoming seriously ill John contacted the woman with whom he had had unprotected sex some months earlier and informed her of his illness. She visited her local GUM clinic and was found to be 'e' antigen positive and, because she had never experienced any symptoms of hepatitis, was a 'silent' hepatitis B carrier. Initially she was unaware of the real significance of this, but after chatting with one of the health advisers she became very distressed when she realised the serious consequences of this diagnosis to her own health, any potential children she might have and other sexual contacts.

After discussion and counselling, John's regular girlfriend was tested and found to be hepatitis B negative and was promptly vaccinated.

References

Alberti, A. (1996) *Clinical gastroenterology*. London: Baillière Tindall.

Alter, H. J. (1996) The cloning and clinical implications of HGV and HGBV-C. *New England Journal of Medicine*; 335: 1536–1537.

Benhamou, J.P., Marcellin, P., Boyer, N. et al (1993) Viral hepatitis. *Gut*; 34: suppl. 2, iv.

Boag, F. (1991) Hepatitis B: heterosexual transmission and vaccination strategies. *International Journal of STDs and AIDS*; 2: 5, 318–324.

British Liver Trust (1996) *Liver Focus* (newsletter); January.

Carlisle, D. (1997) Hepatitis B: is it a disaster waiting to happen? *Health Visitor*; 70: 7, 270–271.

Cowley, H.C., Webster. N. R. (1993) Management of liver disease on ICU. *Care of the Critically Ill*; 9: 3, 122–127.

Curtis, H., Hoolaghan, T., Jewitt, C. (1995) *Sexual Health Promotion in General Practice*. Oxford: Radcliffe Medical Press.

Davison, F., Alexander, G.J.M., Trowbridge, R. et al (1987) Detection of hepatitis B virus DNA in spermatozoa, urine, saliva and leucocytes of chronic HBsAg carriers. *Hepatology*; 4: 1, 37–44.

Deka, N., Sharma, M.D., Mukerjee, R. (1994) Isolation of the novel agent from human stool samples that is associated with sporadic non-A, non-B hepatitis. *Journal of Virology*; 68: 12, 7810–7815.

Department of Health (1993) Protecting health care workers and patients from hepatitis B: recommendations of the Advisory Group on Hepatitis. *HSG*; 93: 40.

Department of Health (1996) *Immunisation Against Infectious Diseases*. London: HMSO.

Edwards, S., Carne. C. (1998) Oral sex and the transmission of viral STIs. *Sexually Transmitted Infections*; 74: 1, 6–10.

Eyster, M.E., Alter, H.J., Aledort, L.M., et al (1991) Heterosexual co-transmission of hepatitis C virus and human immunodeficiency virus (HIV). *Annals of Internal Medicine*; 115: 10, 764–768.

Goldsmith, R., Yarbough, P.O., Reyes, G.R. et al (1992) Enzyme-linked immunosorbent assay for diagnosis of acute sporadic hepatitis E in Egyptian children. *The Lancet*; 339: 341, 328–331.

Group B (1990) *Group B, hepatitis B and you: treatment, vaccines, sex and living with hepatitis*. Group B Materials, London.

Gurevich, I. (1993) Hepatitis part II. Viral hepatitis B, C, and D. *Heart and Lung*; 22: 5, 450–457.

Hart, S. (1990) Guidelines for infection control. *Nursing Standard*; 4: 45, 24–27.

Hep Risk Advisory Board (1996) *Hep risk survey: assessing the awareness, knowledge, exposure to risk activities and attitudes of Europe's 15–25 year olds with respect to hepatitis B*; London: HRAB.

Linnen, J., Wages, J.Jr., Zhang-Keck, Z.Y., et al., (1996) Molecular cloning and disease association of hepatitis G virus: a transfusion-transmissible agent. *Science*; 271: 5248, 505–508.

Lundberg, G.D. (1997) Is hepatitis G virus transmitted sexually? *Journal of American Medical Association*; 277: 532–533.

Mangtani, P, Hall, A.J., Normand C.E. (1995) Hepatitis B vaccination: the cost-effectiveness of alternative strategies in England and Wales. *Journal of Epidemiology and Community Health*; 49: 3, 239–244.

Pujol, F.H., Khudyakov, Y.E., Devesa, M. et al (1998) Hepatitis G virus in Amerindians and other Venezuelan high-risk groups. *Journal of Clinical Microbiology*; 36: 2, 470–474.

Reichard, O., Andersson, J., Schvarcz, R. et al (1991) Ribavirin treatment for chronic hepatitis C. *The Lancet* ; 337: 8749, 1058–1061.

Ross, T., Dickerson. E.J. (1992) Vertical transmission of HIV and HBV. *Maternal and Child Nursing*; 17: 4, 192–195.

Rubio, A., Rey, C., Sanchez-Quijano, A. et al (1997) Is hepatitis G transmitted sexually? *Journal of American Medical Association*; 277: 7, 532–533.

Shorey, J. (1982) Sexually transmitted hepatitis – detection and prevention in both patients and partners. *Consultant*; 22: 173–180.

Skidmore, S.J. (1995) Hepatitis E. *British Medical Journal*; 310, 414–415.

Smith, C., Parle, M., Morris, D.J. (1994) Implementation of government recommendations for immunising infants at risk of hepatitis B. *British Medical Journal*; 309: 1339.

Tedder, R.S., Gilson, R.J., Briggs, M. et al (1991) Hepatitis C virus: evidence for sexual transmission. *British Medical Journal*; 302: 6788, 1229–1302.

Van der Poel C.L., Cuypers, H.T., Reesink, H.W. et al (1991) Confirmation of hepatitis C virus by second generation four-antigen recombinant immunoblot assay and polymerase chain reaction. *The Lancet*; 337: 8737, 317–319.

Vento, S., Garofano, T., Renzini, C. et al (1998) Hepatitis A deadly in hepatitis C sufferers. *New England Journal of Medicine*; 338: 5, 286–290.

WHO (1992) Expanded programme on immunisation. *Weekly Epidemiological Record*; 3: 11–16.

Zuckerman, A.J. (1997a) Prevention of primary liver cancer by immunisation. *New England Journal of Medicine*; 336: 1906–1919.

Zuckerman. A.J. (1997b) *Prevention of hepatitis B in the newborn, children and adolescents*. London: Royal College of Physicians.

13. Gender issues: a historical perspective

Chris McGlynn

Sex is still a subject that is not openly talked about, and sexually transmitted infections (STIs) are talked of even less. As this chapter will look at STIs from an historical perspective the term venereal disease (VD) will sometimes be used, as the literature describing the history uses the term. It will also look particularly at the historical treatment of women.

Traditionally, women have taken the blame for STIs. In the 18th century women identified as prostitutes with syphilis were forced into effective imprisonment in 'lock' hospitals, and were clearly identified by having to wear a yellow dress. During the Second World War a poster campaign warned men to keep away from 'loose, infected women' (Oriel, 1994), who spread venereal disease (a term covering syphilis and gonorrhoea).

There is no evidence to suggest that men were blamed or stigmatised in the same way for having VD. However, the AIDS panic in the 1980s shifted some blame to groups other than women, such as gay men and injecting drug users.

References to STIs can be found as far back as biblical times: 'Washing after copulation, particularly for men with urethral discharge, is mentioned in Leviticus XV' (Davenport-Hines, 1992). When, at the end of the 15th century, syphilis made its first appearance in Europe, it was, according to Quetel (1992), 'a new disease, was more terrifying than leprosy and the plague because of its novelty, its profusion of symptoms, its extreme contagiousness, the suffering it caused and the fact that (in the early years at least) it was often fatal'.

In the 17th century a moralising approach was adopted: 'the temptations of the flesh are to be shunned, and so much the worse for pox sufferers, to treat whom is to simply encourage their lecherous ways' (Quetel, 1992). The English surgeon William Clowes' description of VD as 'pestilent infection of filthy lust' makes his attitude to his patients quite clear (Oriel, 1994).

During the 18th century the emphasis changed from the moral to the medical. The thinking was that 'morality, religious or otherwise, is one thing and disease is another; the pox is a disease and therefore it must be treated' (Quetel, 1992). Mercury was the common treatment.

The physician John Hunter wrote a great deal about syphilis and gonorrhoea, and much has been written in turn about his attempt to prove that syphilis and gonorrhoea were different diseases. This involved a misunderstanding when, in 1767, he was said to have inoculated himself on the glans and foreskin of his penis with pus from a virulent gonorrhoea without realising that the patient from whom he inoculated himself also had syphilis, so from this he deduced that gonorrhoea and syphilis had an identical virus. In other literature it is documented that he didn't, in fact, inoculate himself but medical students.

In 1747 a lock hospital was opened at Hyde Park in London. There are no clear records as to the type of STIs that people were admitted with, but prostitutes and soldiers feature prominently on the patients' list, partly because prostitutes with VD were admitted by force. Blame for infection was firmly attached to prostitutes. Doctors believed that any woman could have 'some taint of venereal disease.' Prostitutes became the main focus of a major panic about morals and public health. While doctors believed it was possible even for virgins to transmit venereal disease, 'it was the prostitute who was the obvious symbol of sexual excess and the easiest target for sexual regulation' (Spongberg, 1997).

In a bid to try and reform them, the prostitutes were expected to pray and undertake acts of penitence in the hospitals. The custom was to make them wear yellow dresses to distinguish them. The conditions in these 'canary wards' were dreadful and the medical care very basic.

In the 19th century syphilis treatment seemed to have reached a standstill, despite the work of Ricord, who distinguished between syphilis and numerous other venereal diseases, notably gonorrhoea. The efficacy of mercury as a treatment was in doubt, but the only other defence that was promoted was the condom.

At about this time academics started to take an interest in syphilis. National and international societies were set up and specialist conferences arranged. Much work was done during the latter part of the 19th century and into the beginning of the 20th century looking at 'microscopic animals' (Oriel, 1992), as interest developed in the micro-organisms that caused venereal disease.

Few women worked in the field of venereal disease, and those who did came to it mainly through their involvement with obstetrics and gynaecology. Oriel (1994) writes about Dame Mary Scharlieb, who worked at The New Hospital for Women (now The Elizabeth Garrett Anderson Hospital) in London as a consultant gynaecologist. She had a keen interest in the effects of venereal diseases on the health and fertility of women. She was also interested in the social aspects and prevention through health and sex education.

It was not until the 1930s that women began to practise in the speciality, often at the beginning of their careers in public health. Their numbers increased during the Second World War, when many servicewomen required specialist treatment. From the 1950s onwards women doctors began to adopt venereology as their first career choice (Oriel, 1994).

The origins of the disease remained attached to women. Spongberg (1997) writes that 'Syphilis and gonorrhoea were largely treated as the product of the diseased female body; the question of male responsibility in the spread of the disease is largely ignored by medical literature ... By the early 19th century all venereal disease appeared to be sexually transmitted by women. Prostitutes became the main focus of a major panic about morals and public health ... Prostitutes came to be seen as not only sexual pariahs, but also as women exhibiting a variety of other forms of deviancy and excess, such as lesbianism, alcoholism and other forms of addiction.'

By pathologising the prostitute, male responsibility for both the sexual exploitation of women and the spread of VD could be conveniently overlooked. There was a lot of debate regarding prostitutes and their control. There were even suggestions that infection should be made a criminal offence.

In 1905 Schaudin and Hoffman made a major breakthrough by identifying a pale-coloured *Treponema* associated with syphilis. In 1910 Ehrlich created salvarsan, also known as '606'. This preparation was the initiation of the treatment of syphilis with arsphenamines, eradicating the use of mercury.

In 1913 there was an outcry in the *British Medical Journal* regarding venereal diseases and the 'conspiracy of silence' surrounding syphilis. In reaction to this a Royal Commission on Venereal Diseases was appointed. It was asked to look at 'the prevalence of venereal diseases in the United Kingdom, their effects on the health of the community, and the means by which those effects could be alleviated or prevented, it being understood that no return to the policy or provisions of the Contagious Diseases Acts of 1864, 1866 or 1869 is to be regarded as falling within the scope of the inquiry'.

The commission consulted surgeons, physicians, paediatricians, eye specialists, pathologists, clergymen and welfare workers, and published its report in 1916. The recommendations became law as the Public Health (Venereal Diseases) Regulations of 1916. The commission was committed to teaching health professionals about venereal diseases, improving the availability of testing facilities and prohibiting the advertising of quack remedies. It also recommended that there should be notification, health education and personal prophylaxis. The notification was outweighed by the need for complete confidentiality – they wanted numbers of cases reported, not names. But Oriel (1994) points out that the commissioners themselves had concerns about educating people to take precautions: 'If it was available, might not a man deliberately fornicate in the knowledge that he would be protected from the consequence of his action?' they asked. This is not dissimilar to the current debate about post-exposure-prophylaxis (PEP), which poses the question: will people put themselves at risk of exposure to HIV knowing they can take these drugs?

There was a major increase in venereal diseases during the First World War, especially within the forces. In 1916 'venereal ablution rooms' were established in all barracks. There the soldiers would wash their genital area, have their urethra irrigated with potassium permanganate solution, and have ointment applied. There were 'packets' of the ointment available and sometimes a condom would be supplied for use as prophylaxis.

In 1917 another report was published by the Royal Commission on Venereal Diseases, one of the recommendations being that 'special clinics for the free and confidential treatment of venereal diseases should be established by local authorities in all large towns, and venereal disease officers appointed to run them' (Oriel, 1994). This caused great angst among many hospital management committees, who did not relish the thought of large numbers of venereal patients attending their hospitals. Consequently, the accommodation was often in an out-of-the-way location, in the basement or at the back of the hospital.

Fear of syphilis was at its height during the inter-war period. Syphilis was rife and propaganda was stepped up: pamphlets, posters, radio, the theatre and the cinema were actively used to frighten people. During the 1920s laboratory services were improved and expanded, and in 1924 a central Venereal Disease Reference Laboratory was established.

The venereal disease services improved with the 1928 Poor Law reforms: 'Many of the old Poor Law Hospitals were upgraded to become municipal hospitals which provided medical care comparable with that of the large voluntary hospitals, and venereal disease clinics shared in the process' (Oriel, 1994). The equipment that was in the clinics didn't alter much between the wars: 'glass syringes for taking blood or giving injections, hypodermic needles (periodically sharpened on a whetstone), a set of urethral sounds and perhaps a urethroscope, and vaginal speculae would all be sterilised on the premises. In addition, most clinics had apparatus for dark-field and light-field microscopy. The intravenous injections of arsenicals needed time and skill, toxic reactions were common, and could be serious, urethral irrigations for urethritis needed care, and complications such as epididymitis and urethral stricture gave many problems' (Oriel, 1994).

The Second World War saw another increase of venereal disease cases. The blame was shifting from prostitutes to 'good-time girls', 'pick-ups', and such like. This was still laying the blame at the woman's feet, but now they 'were not paid by their partners. In truth, their motives were little different from those of the men – a desire for companionship and sex amid the uncertainties of wartime' (Oriel, 1994). Contact tracing was introduced in the USA, and it was tried here with little effect, so 'Defence Regulation 33B' was introduced. This meant that if two men named the same woman, the woman's treatment became mandatory. This system was abandoned in 1947.

In 1948, when the National Health Service came into being, venereal disease management became a national rather than a local responsibility, and venereologists received the appointments, pay and status of physicians and surgeons in other specialities. Penicillin revolutionised the treatment of gonorrhoea and syphilis. The early 1950s saw the introduction of tetracyclines, which were widely used in the treatment of non-specific urethritis, which was not thought to be a particularly serious infection.

In the 1960s there was an increase in STIs. The marked reduction in health education around sexual health, the introduction of the oral contraceptive pill and over-confidence in antibiotics, all contributed to the increase. The increase included other STIs, the so-called 'second generation' infections, such as *Chlamydia trachomatis* and its association with pelvic inflammatory disease (PID).

Genital herpes became prominent in the 1970s, and had a major impact on the anxieties attached to sexual relationships because there was a great deal of media attention and scare-mongering. Genital warts had been around for some time, but there was a major increase in the 1970s. At this time they were seen as little more than unsightly, but for some time now it has been suspected that some strains of wart are associated with cervical cancer. More sophisticated tests were being produced at this time, increasing the workload of the microbiology and virology departments.

In the early 1980s the first cases of human immunodeficiency virus (HIV)/acquired immune deficiency syndrome (AIDS) made their impact. Now, instead of women, it was gay and bisexual men, intravenous drug users (IVDUs) and black Africans who were blamed for the virus. It seems that the group that has escaped blame throughout history is heterosexual men. Perhaps this is the group that should be targeted in future sexual health promotion programmes.

References

Davenport-Hines, R. (1990) *Death and punishment, attitudes to sex in Britain since the Renaissance.* London: Collins Publishing Group.

Oriel, J.D., (1994) *The Scars of Venus, A History of Venereology.* London: Springer-Verlag.

Quetel, C. (1992) *The Pox and Prostitution in the History of Syphilis.* Cambridge: Polity Press.

Spongberg, M. (1997) *Feminising Venereal Disease: The Body of the Prostitute in Nineteenth Century Medical Discourse.* Basingstoke and London: Macmillan Press.

14. Psychosexual issues in sexual health care

Sandy Nelson

OVERVIEW

A person diagnosed with a sexually transmitted infection (STI) rarely feels that it is a simple medical matter. The amount of distress experienced by an individual will relate directly to their understanding of their sexuality, their feelings about the sexual acts involved and the context and relationships these are placed within. Frequently, the dominant concerns for the patients we see are guilt over their own betrayal of a partner or confirmation of a partner's sexual infidelity. Having to expose the details of sexual behaviour to nurses, whom patients may expect to be judgmental, contributes to the anxieties of coming for treatment. These anxieties will affect the person's ability to listen to information given by health care practitioners and will influence whether or not they inform their partner and complete their treatment.

Nurses aim to provide good, non-judgmental care and respond sympathetically and openly to patients, but in the area of sexual health our own judgements and values are constantly challenged and exposed. For example, someone returning regularly to a doctor because of frequent colds is likely to be thought of as unfortunate, whereas someone returning again and again with gonorrhoea is seen as a problem and one that can provoke very powerful emotional reactions on the part of staff. This is inevitable, as sex lies at the heart of intimacy and touches all of us.

Listening to distressed patients can be disturbing and may leave nurses feeling helpless and inadequate. It is tempting, because of this, to retreat behind a more narrow medical model and, consequently, miss the opportunity to help the patient reflect on their relationships and consider changes. However, by being aware of our own values and by listening to each patient as openly as we are able we may make a significant difference to the patient's future sexual health.

Little research has been done into the psychological impact of having a sexually transmitted infection, with the exception of genital herpes and HIV. Phobias about STIs are documented and the impact of having syphilis was recognised but, on the whole, the psychological consequences were not considered important aspects of the management of sexually transmitted infections. Consequently, no clinical psychologists were available in genito-urinary medicine (GUM) clinics and health advisers restricted their role to contact tracing. The availability of reliable, simple treatments was perhaps the reason for the limited interest shown in the psychological effects of diagnoses on patients. The advent of HIV radically altered this and changed the culture in genito-urinary medicine. More consideration was given to the psychological implications of sexually transmitted infections, as an understanding of sexual behaviour became essential in halting the spread of HIV and in supporting people with HIV. This became an even more pertinent concern when research revealed the greater risk of HIV transmission with the co-existence of other STIs (Tuliza et al, 1991).

A large proportion of people affected by STIs tend to be particularly vulnerable members of the population. Reports from several countries, including Britain, Denmark and the USA, indicate that young people with a STI tend to be involved in prostitution, alcoholism and crime and to lead unstable lives in many respects (Birch, 1987). Surveys also suggest a high prevalence of psychological difficulties among GUM clinic attenders. Catalan et al (1981) found 20% of clinic attenders could be described as psychiatric cases. Acute anxiety about having a sexually transmitted infection and awareness of possible exposure to HIV have been related to long-lasting sexual dysfunctions (Cooper, 1988). While it is important to treat such findings with caution, especially as they can increase the stigma associated with STIs, it does suggest that attention to the psychological aspects of STIs may enable patients to receive other help that they require. However, assessing need is no easy matter as high levels of distress are 'normal' responses to infections that continue to bear a stigma.

Despite the attempts of nurses working in sexual health to promote a positive approach to sexuality and openness to the diversity of sexual expression, the general culture remains negative about sex. In a recent study of university students (Moore et al, 1995) attitudes to STIs were more negative than to other, non-sexual medical conditions. 'Ashamed', 'unclean' and 'degraded' were the adjectives associated with these infections. Research into young people's attitudes to safer sex shows how condom use can be negotiated as a method of birth control but not as a means of preventing the transmission of STIs (Holland et al, 1998). To argue for condom use to guard against the risk of infection is seen as insulting to the partner and distrusting of them. Given these prevailing attitudes, having a sexually transmitted infection is likely to elicit feelings of being dirty and ashamed, guilty and disgusted.

Although many young men, as well as women, feel mortified to find out they have a sexually transmitted infection, gender plays a significant part in how individuals make sense of their diagnosis. For some young men, having a STI is something to be proud of as they see it as public evidence of their sexual prowess. A doctor in a public health centre in a large city in the USA states: 'They can't wait to go down and show the guys the green drip in their underwear when they're in the gym. They laugh about it, it's a riot! You see kids twelve, thirteen, fourteen, and this is great, it shows they're a real man.' (Hudson and Ineichen, 1991).

Young people often blame the woman for transmitting the infection, with both boys and girls controlling female sexual expression through describing girls as either 'nice' girls or 'slags'. In this context, requests that someone inform their sexual partners about having a sexually transmitted infection and comply with safer sex guidelines while being treated, present complex challenges to those involved. Valued relationships may be placed at risk and disclosure can lead to physical violence as well as verbal abuse, the acquisition of a 'reputation' or the loss of a relationship, so it is not surprising that young people may prefer the risk of constant reinfection to jeopardising their relationships or, for the young men described above, may prefer to exploit the regular infections as badges of honour rather than of shame.

At the other end of the spectrum, many patients experience having a STI as a misfortune rather than a trauma. Nevertheless, whether they find their condition deeply humiliating or a minor inconvenience, each patient will have had to come to terms with it in the context of the values of the groups with which they identify. Age, ethnicity, gender, sexual orientation, friendships, partners and geographical location will all influence their understanding of their infection. A poignant example of this was the statement by a black African woman requesting a repeat HIV test as she could not believe the positive result she had been given: 'I'm good and you only get HIV when you are bad, black and poor'.

Patients' responses to their diagnoses will elicit varied reactions from staff. Nurses often ruefully acknowledge that, when faced with a distraught woman feeling that no-one will ever love her again, they will emphasise that STIs can be caught by anyone sexually active, whereas they will outline as vividly as possible the potential long-term consequences to a man indifferent to the welfare of his partners and refusing to consider safer sex as it would interfere with his pleasure. A similar picture emerges from McCrombie's (1986) study into the counselling given to 'high-risk' and 'low-risk' individuals requesting HIV tests – she noted that regardless of the actual HIV result, 'high-risk' individuals were 'chastised, admonished and warned', whereas 'low-risk' individuals were 'consoled and reassured'. This demonstrates how easy it is to convey moral judgments despite attempting not to.

Sexual history taking and genital examinations can enable patients to explore aspects of their sexuality previously hidden or denied. Genital examinations are known to be powerful triggers for memories of sexual abuse or assault. In the confidential and anonymous environment of the GUM clinic patients can acknowledge psychosexual problems. Gay men, in particular, may feel that the GUM environment is more open to their sexual orientation and may feel it is possible to reveal a psychosexual problem without the problem being seen as their homosexuality itself. The crisis of discovering the presence of a STI can bring about a reassessment of current behaviour and can lead some patients to be particularly receptive to discussions about the risks taken and how they might be minimised. The potential to support patients in their explorations and to refer appropriately when necessary is an important part of the management of STIs.

One of the difficulties in researching the psychological effect of STIs is the range of conditions these cover. The emotional response to bacterial vaginosis, for instance, will be very different from the response to HIV. Obviously, this is because HIV involves questions of mortality, potential long-term illness which will require extensive medical management, possible disfigurement (with Karposi's sarcoma which, distressing in itself, also publicly signals one's HIV status), contagiousness to sexual partners and infection by a virus that continues to be highly stigmatised. The impact of other STIs will depend to a certain extent on how many of these factors pertain. However, it will also depend on the previous psychological well being of the person involved and sometimes even minor infections can be difficult for some people to manage. The physical symptoms can be quickly and successfully cleared up, but the crisis in relationships can take much longer to heal.

It is easy to underestimate the distress that may be experienced. Genital warts, for instance, are such a common condition that the psychological effects can easily be ignored. Yet its association with cancer, the possibility of recurrence and the long incubation period make some patients feel that they will be unable to have a sexual relationship again. Cervical smear tests are another example of something so routine to women's sexual health care that the anxiety related to them can be overlooked. Confusion about the meaning of having mild or moderate dyskaryotic smear results and the misunderstanding that these mean they have cancer can create enormous distress for the women involved. If further tests and treatments are required they can be a source of much worry and uncertainty.

Many patients have difficulty coping with the limitations of our knowledge regarding the transmission of many STIs. They wish to have precise facts that are not available. Lesbians, in particular, often get confusing and conflicting advice about how to protect their sexual partners. One study indicated considerable inconsistency in the risk assessments given by staff for various sexual activities, with oral sex being a particular area of difficulty. Inevitably, this increases the bewilderment and anxiety levels felt by patients as they struggle to make sense of the information they are given. It is a complex problem as, although it is vital that nurses are honest about risks and do not minimise them, if people feel that safer sex is too demanding they may not consider it.

Ensuring that patients have adequate information to take away with them is an important part of helping them manage their anxieties. Women undergoing cytological investigations related their satisfaction to the quality of the explanation received (Bell et al, 1995), indicating how essential this educative aspect of the work is. Yet this is a deceptively difficult task as most verbal information is forgotten (Ley, 1979). Patients often fail to understand the information they are given and situations with high levels of anxiety impede the ability to absorb information. Criticism has been levelled at HIV pre-test counselling, claiming that it can be over-burdened with information and advice giving (Bond, 1990). Leaflets, therefore, can be useful when anxieties are high. However, the quality of leaflets available is very varied. Marteau et al (1996) found that pamphlets provided for women attending for colposcopies had very different effects on the women reading them: those that gave complex information did nothing to alleviate anxiety, whereas those that were written more simply and that contained strategies for coping were far more useful.

HERPES SIMPLEX VIRUS

More research has been done into the psychological impact of having genital herpes simplex virus than other sexually transmitted infections (HIV is considered separately). The amount of distress this virus can cause is very familiar to anyone working in GUM. The fact that it is likely to recur, that it can be extremely painful and debilitating and that the sores are on the most intimate part of the body, all contribute to the distress caused. Previously, people with herpes could be reassured that they were only infectious to partners when symptomatic, but more recent evidence of transmission when asymptomatic (Cunningham et al, 1997) means that they are placed in the position of having to disclose that they have herpes to new partners or risk transmitting the infection to them. Because it is a lifelong problem it emerges as an issue whenever a new sexual relationship is begun and profoundly changes people's self-image – one woman said she felt as if she had 'a big H' on her forehead, another that it felt like a big germ (Pyett, 1995). Others commented that the emotional aspect of herpes is the most difficult to cope with. One young woman stated: 'the pain of it ... is horrible. But it's not a stitch on what it does to your nervous system emotionally.' (Pyett, 1995).

Most patient's reported shame, guilt, feeling dirty, isolated and unable to talk to others about it (Pyett, 1995). Depression, anger and reduced self-confidence were common (Drob et al, 1985). The fears of rejection are not unfounded – according to Reiser (1986) many people in his study reported that they would end a relationship if their partner had herpes.

Despite this, many people are able to manage a diagnosis of herpes perfectly well. Previous functioning, levels of self-esteem and the strength of current relationships will, to a large extent, determine the individual's response to it. Some people use it as an opportunity to make positive changes. Others, already more fragile, use it to retreat from sexual relationships and isolate themselves from others.

Although there are differences, many of these findings are likely to apply to other STIs. Stronks (1993) found little difference in the psychological consequences of herpes and gonorrhoea. Self-blame is found as a common reaction in research into nearly all STIs.

HIV

Anyone who has a sexually transmitted infection has simultaneously placed themselves at risk of contracting HIV. It is likely that this will be an anxiety for most people diagnosed with other STIs, therefore it is important to consider, at least briefly, the psychological implications of HIV. In addition, much that we have come to understand about HIV may well apply to other STIs despite important differences.

Choosing to have an HIV test is often the result of some personal crisis or has symbolic importance for the individual. Some people come for tests with partners to signify their commitment to one another and their decision to stop practising safer sex if they are both negative; others come because they suspect infidelity or because they have had an affair or visited a prostitute and feel guilty and ashamed. Some come because of anxiety about risks they have taken in the past. Others come because they have other STIs or symptoms that doctors think may be HIV-related. Even people who believe their risks are low worry about the result. Waiting for the result can be an extremely difficult period. The window period extends the agony, and the introduction of condom use, or abstinence from sexual intercourse, may precipitate crises in relationships. Yet this is also a time when people reassess their sexual practices and, through acknowledging their vulnerability to infection, strengthen commitment to changes in behaviour. Many, in fact, seek out an HIV test because they are already considering changes they wish to make.

One group of people, referred to as the 'worried well' come regularly for HIV tests. The 'worried well' are people who are convinced they are HIV positive despite negative test results. They are suffering and do need help, but they can be difficult and frustrating to work with as they are often unwilling to acknowledge a psychological basis for their fears. This group contains people with a broad range of problems and by listening to their fears it may be possible to work out what function the worry about HIV is serving for them. Questions about what was going on for them when the fears began, current relationship difficulties and past psychiatric history may suggest likely causes and help nurses to make appropriate referrals.

Attempts to reassure patients about their negative status are futile as this merely reinforces the problem. Instead, it is necessary to try to get them to accept the psychological basis for their problem. This is not an easy thing to do, but can be helped by avoiding being drawn into a discussion of HIV and by focusing instead on the anxiety of the patient and ways (other than testing) they might deal with it.

A positive HIV result will change the lives of all those infected. Their perception of themselves will change as they come to terms with what being a person with HIV means to them. No matter how much they may have anticipated a positive result, confirmation is a shock. As well as facing their own mortality, they have to consider disclosing the information to partners, family and friends and contemplate what the reaction will be to their HIV status – will people close to them be supportive?

Many people infected are refugees from countries at war, who have already had multiple losses, faced torture, violence and the loss of their homeland and community. Some will have struggled with problems related to drug use; others have issues regarding their sexuality. All of these will affect their response to HIV and their ability to cope with a diagnosis. Suicide attempts may be feared, and in order to enable nurses to judge the risk it is important to find out about any previous suicide attempts and to assess what support a patient will have from friends and family.

In contrast, some people feel that having HIV has enabled them to make positive changes in their lives. For most it is a mixture of good and bad, with periods of depression and desperation followed by times of well-being and hope. Nevertheless, however an individual comes to terms with their diagnosis it will involve considerable and continual emotional work – difficult decisions regarding treatments will have to be faced, people close to them may die and they have to learn to live with the multiple changes brought about through having HIV.

SEXUAL ASSAULT AND ABUSE

Giving a sexual history, having a genital examination, receiving a diagnosis of a STI and undergoing pre-test counselling for HIV can all trigger traumatic memories related to previous sexual experiences. Having the opportunity to talk about sexuality may enable people to talk about previously buried experiences. Nurses who have been sexually assaulted or abused themselves may find working with these patients particularly difficult. Even when this is not the case these patients can be particularly distressing to work with. Through discussion with a clinical supervisor or trusted colleague nurses can explore their anxieties about this work and formulate strategies in advance to support both themselves and patients.

Sexual abuse and assault both result in short- and long-term trauma that will be mediated by the experience itself and all the other factors that affected it, such as its duration, the age at which it occurred and the relationship with the abuser. The patient's support network and current stresses will also be relevant. By assessing these factors different kinds of help may be suggested, from crisis intervention through to long-term therapy.

Many people assaulted come in for screening soon after the event has occurred, often because it has been recommended. Despite their distress, at this time only a few wish to talk over what has happened. For those who fear talking about it and wish to forget it and get on with their lives as quickly as possible leaflets can help considerably. Often people superficially come to terms with the assault and then find themselves having nightmares, panic attacks or difficulty with sleeping and eating. The leaflets can provide reassurance that these are normal reactions. For those who do wish to talk, staff need to receive training on how to support these patients. Nurses can feel under enormous pressure as they try to listen to the person who has been assaulted and yet feel inadequately trained and unsure of how to respond. Conflict can also be felt because of the other patients waiting for attention. Structures specifically for these patients need to be set up to support both the nurse and the person who has been sexually assaulted. These structures, however, can only help with those patients who identify themselves as attending because of sexual assault, and do not help when the trigger is unexpected. These 'out of the blue' reactions can be the hardest to deal with and to understand. It may be as shocking for the patient as it is for the nurse when carefully constructed defences are stripped away.

Both abuse and assault can lead to sexual problems and can make medical examinations intolerable. Men who have been assaulted may find disclosure difficult because of shameful feelings of not being a 'real' man. Shame for both men and women makes disclosure hard and many have difficulty labelling what happened to them as assault. Similarly, people who have been assaulted, and those around them, readily dismiss as trivial assault that has not involved actual penetration or violence. Yet the amount of trauma experienced is associated more with the level of fear and anticipation of death or injury than the actual event. Sensitive explorations of these issues can enable patients to assess their situation and decide if the assault or abuse is affecting their current lives in ways that would make it appropriate to seek further help.

EFFECT ON THE HEALTH CARE WORKER

By allowing ourselves to think about the differing emotional responses we have to patients we may be able to understand more about the patient's inner world. These responses are often far removed from ideals we may hold of the good nurse because they can involve disgust, fury and uncomfortably strong and sometimes disturbing feelings.

Ethical dilemmas involving confidentiality, the age of patients, behaviours that are destructive to the self and others can provoke conflicting feelings. In particular, nurses can find the maintenance of confidentiality distressing. Knowing that someone you are seeing is being lied to by their partner about the sexual behaviour they are engaged in can be hard to bear and can arouse feelings of anger, protectiveness and righteous indignation that have to be managed by the nurse while outwardly adhering to confidentiality policies. Patient's failures to comply with treatments, inform partners who may be infected, change behaviours that put others at risk and take risks that deliberately place themselves at risk put an enormous burden on the nurse. Clinical supervision is a crucial support for practitioners faced with these issues.

We know through our own experiences in sexual health clinics that people continually return, having been reinfected with a STI. Research supports this, demonstrating that previous STIs have no impact on subsequent preventive practices (O'Campo et al, 1992; Fullilove et al, 1990). The nurse's agenda can be irrelevant or even the opposite of the patient's, and the patient's beliefs about how they have come to be infected may be entirely different to those of the nurse, with some women, for example, not attributing their infection to sexual behaviour at all (Redfern and Hutchinson, 1994). Other research records the voices of six young African Americans who seroconverted after deliberately exposing themselves to HIV. Their descriptions of their sense of utter futility and hopelessness living with gang warfare, violence, drug abuse and minimal opportunities for escape link their 'choice' of HIV with the destructiveness surrounding them (Tourigny, 1998). Other studies indicate that risking unsafe sex amongst young gay men is related to feelings of low self-esteem (Gold and Skinner, 1992).

All of this forces us to confront the complexity of sexual behaviour and relationships, and requires us to try and understand the inner lives of those we encounter. It is only by listening to the person's own story that we may be able to offer relevant and appropriate support. Staff development, training and clinical supervision are all required to enable nurses to provide care which addresses the psychological issues that are such a fundamental aspect of sexual health care.

References

Bell, S., Porter, M., Kichener, H., et al (1995) Psychological response to cervical screening. *Preventive Medicine*; 246, 610–616.

Birch, D.M.L. (1987) *Are you my sister Mummy?* London: Youth Support.

Bond, T. (1991) *HIV Counselling*. Rugby: British Association for Counselling.

Catalan, J., Bradley, M., Gallwey, J. et al (1981) Sexual dysfunction and psychiatric morbidity in patients attending a clinic for sexually transmitted diseases. *British Journal of Psychiatry*; 138, 292–296.

Cooper, G. F. (1988) The psychological methods of sex therapy. In Cole, M., Dryden, W (eds.) *Sex Therapy in Britain*. Milton Keynes: Open University Press.

Cunningham, A.L., Flexman, J.P., Dwyer, D. et al (1997) *Clinicians' Manual on Genital Herpes*. London: Science Press.

Drob, S., Loemer, M., Lifshutz, H. (1985) Genital herpes: the psychological consequences. *British Journal of Medical Psychology*; 58, 307–315.

Fullilove, R.E., Fullilove, M.T., Bowser, B.P. (1990) Risk of sexually transmitted disease among black adolescent crack users in Oakland and San Francisco, California. *Journal of the American Medical Association*; 263, 851–855.

Gold, R.S., Skinner, M.J. (1992) Situational factors and thought processes associated with unprotected intercourse in young gay men. *AIDS Journal*; Sept 01: 6, 1021–1030.

Holland, J., Ramazanoglu, C., Sharpe, S. et al (1998) *The male in the head: young people, heterosexuality and power*. London: The Tufnell Press.

Ley, P. (1979) Memory for Medical Information. *British Journal of Social and Clinical Psychology*; 18, 245–255.

Hudson, F., Ineichen, B. (1991) *Taking it Lying Down: Sexuality and Teenage Motherhood*. Basingstoke: Macmillan.

Marteau, T.M., Kidd, J., Cuddeford, L. et al (1996) Reducing anxiety in women referred for colposcopy using an information booklet. *British Journal of Health Psychology*; 1: 2, 181–189.

Montford, H., Skrine, R. (1993) *Contraceptive Care*. London: Chapman & Hall.

Moore, S. Rosenthal, D. Mitchell, A. (1996) *Youth, AIDS and Sexually Transmitted Diseases*. London: Routledge.

O'Campo, P., Deboer, M., Faden, R.R. et al (1992) Prior episode of sexually transmitted disease and subsequent risk reduction interventions. *Sexually Transmitted Diseases*; 19, 326–230.

Pyett, P. (1995) *Living with Herpes: A report to the Melbourne Herpes Self-Help Group (HELM)*. Melbourne: Centre for the Study of Sexually Transmissible Diseases, La Trobe University.

Redfern, N., Hutchinson, S. (1994) Women's experiences of repeatedly contracting sexually transmitted diseases. *Health Care for Women International*; 15: 5, 423–433.

Reiser, C. (1986) Herpes: a physical and moral dilemma. *College Student Journal*; 20: 260–269. In Moore, S. et al (1996) *Youth, AIDS and Sexually Transmitted Diseases*. London: Routledge.

Stronks, D.L., Rijpma, S.E., Passchier, J., et al (1993) Psychological consequences of genital herpes, an exploratory study with a gonorrhoea control group. *Psychological Reports*; 73: 2, 395–400.

Tourigny, S.C. (1998) Some new dying trick: African American youth 'choosing' HIV/AIDS. *Qualitative Health Research*; 8: 2, 149–167, March.

Tuliza, M., Manoka, A.T., Nzila, N., et al (1991) The impact of STD control and condom promotion on the incidence of HIV in Kinshasa prostitutes (Abstract MC 3061). *Seventh International Conference on AIDS*; Florence, June 1991.

Index